CW01304414

We dedicate this book to those who are alone and who suffer loneliness, stress, anxiety, and depression.

Feel Better In 70 Seconds™

Help Beat Depression and Feel Better With 10 Easy to Perform Exercises For a Total-Body Workout With Scientifically Proven Isometrics

Published by
MajorVision International
2020

Approved by The World Isometric Exercise Association
www.TWiEA.com

TWiEA
The World Isometric Exercise Association

Copyright and Trademark Notice
© 2020 Brian Sterling-Vete and Helen Renée Wuorio All Rights Reserved

All material in this book is the property of, copyright, and trademarked to Brian Sterling-Vete and Helen Renée Wuorio, and/or MajorVision Ltd unless otherwise stated, AE&OE. Copyright and other intellectual property laws protect these materials. Reproduction, distribution, or transmission of the materials, in whole or in part, in any manner, without the prior written consent of the copyright holder is prohibited and is a violation of national and international copyright law.

The following names, exercises, and workout systems are the property of, copyright, and trademarked to Brian Sterling-Vete, Helen Renée, and/or MajorVision Ltd. ISOfitness™, The 70 Second Difference™, Adaptive Response™, Zero Footprint Workout™, Fitness on the Move™, FOM™, The ISO90™ Course, ISO90™, The SSASS Workout™, SSASS™, Dynamic Flexation™, The Bullworker Bible™, The Bullworker 90™, The Bullworker Compendium™, Workout at Work™, Doorway to Strength™, The TRISO90™ Course, TRISOmetrics™, The ISOmetric Bible™, Brian Sterling-Vete's Mental Martial Arts™, Tuxedo Warriors™, Being American Married to a Brit™, Paranormal Investigation - The Black Book of Scientific Ghost Hunting and How to Investigate Paranormal Phenomena™, The Haunting of Lilford Hall™, Isometric Exercises for Nordic Walking and Trekking™ Pt.1 & 2, Isometric Power Exercises for Martial Arts™, Isometric Exercises for Golf Pt.1 & 2™, Isometric Exercises for Scuba Diving Pt.1 & 2™, The Zero-Footprint Lockdown Workout™, Feel Better In 70 Seconds™.

Artwork, designed by MAJORVISION.COM

Contents

Important General Safety and Health Guidelines

1. **The World Changed**
   - A Little Can Mean a Lot
   - A Broken Heart Can Kill You
   - Anxiety
   - Depression
   - Mental Health and Exercise
   - Depression, Mood and Exercise
   - The 70 Second Difference™
   - 21 Days to a New Habit?

2. **Exercise Science Overview**
   - The Basic Types of Resistance Exercise
   - Isometric Overview
   - Isometric Exercise Science
   - The Standard Isometric Contraction
   - Workout Intensity
   - Technically, How Does a Muscle Grow?
   - Rest Time Between Exercises
   - Dynamic Flexation™
   - Isometric Exercises and Blood Pressure
   - Rest and Recovery
   - Adequate Nutrition is Vital

3. **Isometric Exercise Tools**
   - Improvised Isometric Exercise Devices
     - Rope – Either Climbing Rope or Towing Rope
     - The Humble Beach or Bath Towel
     - The Broom Handle
     - The Walking Stick/Pole
   - Proprietary Isometric Exercise Equipment

- Securing the Iso-Bow® With Your Feet
4. **How Effective is a 10x7 Second Total-Body Workout? And About the Exercise Model**
5. **Things to Remember Before You Begin**
    - The Essential Feel Better in 70 Seconds 10x7 Second Exercise Workout Routine Overview
6. **The Feel Better in 70 Seconds 10x7 Second Exercise Workout Routine**
    - 1) Abdominal Knee Raise and Trunk Curl
    - 2 & 3) Biceps and Triceps Dual Self-Resistance (Left and Right Side)
        - Variation Arms: Biceps and Triceps Dual Resistance with Rope
        - Variation Arms: Biceps and Triceps Dual Resistance with Iso-Bow®- Long Bow
        - Variation Arms: Biceps and Triceps Dual Resistance with Iso-Bow® - Short Bow
    - 4) Back: Upper Chest-Level Pull-Apart
        - Variation Upper Back: Pull-Apart with Rope
        - Variation Upper Back: Pull-Apart with Towel
        - Variation Upper Back: Pull-Apart Iso-Bow®
    - 5) Lower Back: Lying Shoulder and Legs Raise
        - Variation Lower Back: Deadlift with Rope
    - 6) Chest: Palm-Press Together

- Variation Chest: Press Together with Rope Looped Around Hands
- Variation Chest: Press Together with Iso-Bow®
▲ 7) Shoulders: Side Lateral Raise Hands Interlock
- Variation Shoulders: Side Lateral Raise with Rope
- Variation Shoulders: Side Lateral Raise with Towel
- Variation Shoulders: Side Lateral Raise with Iso-Bow®
- Variation Shoulders: Side Lateral Raise with Rope Under Feet
▲ 8) Upper Thighs Front: Wall Squat
- Variation Upper Thighs Front: Squat with Rope
▲ 9) Upper Thigh Hamstring: Wall Hamstring Curl
▲ 10) Calf: Immovable Object Heel Raise-Push

7. **Conclusion**
   ▲ What is TWiEA™?

Important General Safety and Health Guidelines

This section entitled, "Important General Safety and Health Guidelines," pertains to The ISOfitness™ Exercise System, and all books and publications about it not limited to but including The ISO90™ Course, Fitness on the Move™, The 70 Second Difference™, The Bullworker Bible™, The Sixty Second Ass Workout™, The Bullworker 90™ Course, The Bullworker Compendium™, Workout at Work™, The Doorway to Strength™, TRISOmetrics™, The TRISO90™ Course, the TRISOmetric™ system, The ISOmetric Bible™, Isometric Power Exercises for Martial Arts™, Isometric Exercises for Nordic Walking and Trekking™ Parts 1 and 2., Isometric Exercises for Golf™ Parts 1 and 2., Isometric Exercises for Scuba Diving™ Parts 1 and 2, The Zero Footprint Lockdown Workout™, Feel Better In 70 Seconds™ general and specific recommendations, suggestions, coaching, and advice, either written, verbal, in audio format, on video, written, or given, implied, or suggested the authors, from Brian Sterling-Vete, Helen Renée Wuorio, and the works thereof.

You should never begin any kind of sport, exercise system, workout plan, or diet modification, including everything contained in this book and in any books mentioned in the beginning paragraph above unless you have consulted with and have the full approval of your medical doctor.

Your physician can accurately assess your current health status, and your ability to perform the exercises in the book and/or course. This is particularly important if you have any known or unknown pre-existing health issues, if you are pregnant, or if you believe that you may have other serious health conditions.

You must always have the absolute approval from your physician/GP before starting. Please show all the material in the above courses, books, video/audio, online material, and their content to your physician and get their approval before you start.

All exercises, suggestions, recommendations, instructions, exercise plans, dietary and eating recommendations, either given or implied, are intended only as a reference, and they are no substitute for a qualified professional personal coach who can help you to plan an exercise and diet program appropriate for your age and physical condition. Never overexert yourself when performing any exercise.

Stop exercising immediately and always either consult your doctor and/or call the EMS immediately if you ever experience any pain, irregular heartbeat, shortness of breath, tightness in your chest/arms/fingers, faintness, nausea, or feelings of dizziness.

The exercises, courses, plans, and dietary recommendations in this book together with all those mentioned in all the books, general publications, online material, and videos mentioned in the names in paragraph 1 of this section, are not intended for use by children. Keep all exercise equipment out of the reach of children.

Always inspect any exercise equipment, and/or any/all other improvised or specifically made exercise equipment/materials, doors, door jambs, and door frames, and anything else you use before each use to ensure its proper operation and to ensure that it is undamaged and safe. Do not use it unless all parts are free from wear, and it is functioning properly.

To avoid serious injury, care should always be taken using any/all exercise equipment, and in all items, people, books, and courses, mentioned in paragraph 1 of this section.

Care should always be taken when getting into all exercise positions, on and off the floor, on and off chairs, on and off benches, on and off any other surface that might be used for exercise, including pieces of furniture, and in the use of all exercised equipment, either purpose-made or improvised.

The creators, writers, instructors, originators, and owners of The Bullworker 90™ Course, The TRISO 90™ Course, The ISO 90™ Course, and all other courses/books, publications on video, audio, and in print, together with the courses, and websites, owned, originated, and created by the copyright holders and the ISOfitness™ and TWiEA™ team, including, but not limited to all books, courses, and people mentioned in paragraph 1 of this section, accept no responsibility whatsoever for any injury, harm, damage, illness, harm, damage to property, or any other negative health-related condition which may occur as a direct, or indirect result of following these courses, recommendations, suggestions, diagrams, pictures, videos, or while performing any exercises in these or any related other related material/publication/s.

For additional general information, we also recommend that you check reputable accredited medical advice sites such as the two listed here. The National

Health Service in the United Kingdom, online at: https://www.nhs.uk/Livewell/fitness/pages/physical-activity-guidelines-for-adults.aspx

In the USA, The Mayo Clinic online: http://www.mayoclinic.org/healthy-lifestyle/fitness/in-depth/exercise/art-20047414

Chapter 1: The World Changed

In the early Spring of 2020, the world changed forever. This was not because of Brexit, or a general election, or because of Harry and Meghan were making fools of themselves again at every possible opportunity, or anything else essentially superficial and sensationalist like that. Instead, it was because of an invisible enemy that was killing people.

Newsfeeds began to carry stories about a deadly new virus that had somehow taken hold in a city in China and was killing a lot of people because we had no current medicine that could combat it. Incidentally, I should mention now that I am not actually allowed to state the obvious and name the virus. This is because if I do then amazingly, this publishing platform will not allow me to publish this book. So, from this point onwards since thoughts are being policed, I will simply refer to it from now on as the GGV, or Great Global Virus.

Gradually, the same newsfeeds began to carry more traffic about how this virus was beginning to spread from the source city and gradually spread across China and outwards from there. Unfortunately, the mainstream media has become its own worst enemy. For many, ourselves included, the mainstream media has completely lost credibility, so, very few people took the news about the virus too seriously. After all, why should they? Let us face it, barely a year has gone by in the last 20 years or so when the mainstream media have not carried shock headlines about some new kind of supposedly killer virus. A virus that is so deadly that there is no stopping it and how very soon we are all going to end up living out the rest of our lives in the dystopia of some kind of badly made B-movie about zombies. In short, the mainstream media had cried *wolf* once too often to be taken seriously.

However, for once the media were right. There was a deadly virus, we had no known medicine that could combat it and it was spreading like wildfire across the globe. The problem was that because the media had cried *wolf* once too often people and even governments across the globe were complacent and slow to act. This allowed the virus to take hold and spread faster than anyone ever imagined.

It is uncanny how in 1720 there was the last major outbreak of bubonic plague in western Europe which came to be known as The Great Plague of Marseille. Around 100 years after that, between 1817 and 1824, the first cholera pandemic began near the city of Calcutta and spread throughout Southeast Asia to the Middle East, eastern Africa, and the Mediterranean coast. Again, after around another 100 years, between 1918 and 1920 there was a pandemic of Spanish Flu, which is around 100 years before the Great Global Virus pandemic of 2020. Do not forget, I am not allowed to call it by its real name.

The Spanish flu pandemic lasted from January 1918 to December 1920 and it infected approximately 500 million people which was about a quarter of the world's population at the time. Suddenly, people began to remember their history lessons about this and comparing it to the GGV pandemic that was only just beginning. People became terrified because the Spanish Flu is estimated to have killed between 17 million and 50 million, with some experts estimating that the actual death toll could have been as high as 100 million. There was no mistaking the fact that the Spanish Flu pandemic was of the deadliest in human history.

Medicine of the time was by modern standards archaic. Even though this was only 100 years ago, it may as well have been the Dark Ages. In 1918, doctors had almost nothing of any real value which they could use to effectively treat Spanish Flu with, and all they could do was to try and alleviate some of the effects. However, they did their best, and with good intentions, but they may have even done more harm than good at times. In 2009, a paper published in the journal called *Clinical Infectious Diseases*, Karen Starko proposed that aspirin poisoning may have significantly contributed to many of the Spanish Flu deaths. This is because the Journal of the American Medical Association and the Surgeon General of the U.S. Army at the time both recommended the administration of what we now know to be dangerous doses of aspirin. They recommended that doses of between 8 and 31 grams of aspirin should be administered per day to treat the disease. The problem with that is this sort of dosage will cause around 3% of patients to suffer lung oedema and up to 33% of patients to hyperventilate. Neither of these scenarios can be any good to someone suffering the already severe symptoms of Spanish Flu.

The only saving grace in 2020 was that science had progressed significantly since those times. In comparison, the science of 1918 may as well have been using stone knives, trepanation (boring holes in the skull), mercury tonics, leeches to bleed people with and animal dung ointments. Incidentally, all the things I just mentioned were real treatments administered by so-called medical doctors at some time in history. Patients of the time may as well have consulted their pet dog for all the good these treatments did them. In 2020, we may not exactly have progressed to the levels of medical science aboard the Starship Enterprise, but it had progressed far enough to offer some serious treatment options and even several vaccine choices too.

To help prevent the spread of the GGV in 2020, most sensible governments immediately implemented an emergency lockdown of people on a national scale. This was the most severe peacetime curtailing of people's freedoms together with social and work habits that had ever been set into place. The entire populations of Britain, most European countries, and many parts of the United States were told categorically by respective governments and the World Health Organisation to "Stay at home indoors or risk dying", and most did. Naturally, there are always some idiots who believe the rules do not apply to them, or that somehow, they always know better, but by and large most sensible people complied with the new rules.

As we write this book, we are in week three of the self-isolation lockdown at our home in April 2020. We are lucky because my wife and I have each other. We also have a fantastic 4-year-old greyhound companion who loves a morning sprint once or twice around the apartment complex where we live, and then to settle down and watch a John Wayne movie. Yes, as strange as it may sound our dog really does love to watch John Wayne movies and he will sprawl out on the sofa for hours on end watching The Duke's movies on a spare laptop we leave just for him.

We may have to maintain appropriate social distancing during essential travel for food, and despite the glorious sunshine and balmy weather of spring we are not allowed to travel to beaches of the countryside, we still have an incredibly good life. We have plenty of laughs each day, a whacky, characterful dog, and we are also able to exercise regularly with isometrics just as if nothing had changed. The strange thing is though, that even though we have all these wonderful things, life still seems to be a little bleaker. Somehow, we still feel alone to a certain degree. It still somehow feels more like survival than we are living life. Sometimes, it has felt a little like we are living our version of the movie *Castaway* starring Tom Hanks.

Millions of people all over the world were all doing the same thing and self-isolating at home. This also means that at the time of writing this book, more people than ever in the history of the world are now living alone. However, a huge number of people do not have a partner, or a dog, a friendly neighbourhood, or anything else like that. Many do not even have a TV, a DVD player, a laptop, a modern cellular phone, or even something as simple as a nice view form, their lounge window. They have nothing except isolation.

Herein lie some of the dangers that will be the equally deadly fallout of the 2020 pandemic. Research has shown that isolation, stress, and anxiety have a serious cascade effect on the brain and body. People are beginning to feel increasingly vulnerable to the virus. This is just like the bogeyman under the bed scenario when we are children. How our perspective shifts and distorts as the minutes pass in the darkness of our bedroom. How we feel increasingly vulnerable as we believe that every creak and groan of the house is actually the bogeyman under the bed, and not just our parents getting ready for bed in the other room. This is only a tiny glimpse of isolation anxiety, but it still caused our hearts to race as we shook in fear hidden under our bedsheets.

For all those millions of people who are all alone dealing with the enforced self-isolation together the ever-looming spectre of the killer virus stalking us, this is a real-life bogeyman scenario. Millions will be suffering the resultant higher blood pressure, increased levels of cortisol (the stress hormone) which helps to cause inflammation.

One of the world's leading researchers in this field is Julianne Holt-Lunstad, a psychologist at Brigham Young University and a fellow of the Society of Experimental Social Psychology and Association for Psychological Science. Her research has estimated that living alone, general social isolation, and loneliness carried the toll of around a 30% mortality rate. I have rounded up the figures which were within a percent or two of each other. These figures are now simply alarming because millions of people are now living all alone and more isolated than ever before during the pandemic lockdown.

Even after the pandemic lockdown is over, to some degree there will be an imprinted after-effect on everyone. The damage may last a lifetime and the dangers too. for example, my parents lived through World War 2. Therefore, even after the war they tended to hoard food, they rarely threw anything away and always stored blankets, candles, matches and other wartime-like essential supplies. Holocaust survivors tended to hoard food long after the war was over and even though they were safe and well living in Great Britain of the USA. The hoarding list could go on to fill several pages alone.

For those who lived through World War 2, there was also the imprint of trauma to live with long after the war had ended. This was not just restricted to those who served in the military because, in Great Britain, everyone was on the frontline each evening as darkness fell. This was when thousands of bombs fell on British cities from the German bombers during the blitz.

In those days, my grandparents had a famous pub near the centre of Manchester where my mother worked helping behind the bar. One evening a German bomb fell on what was then All Saints Church on Oxford Road. It completely obliterated it, and the blast was so massive that it blew up the attached cemetery sending countless pieces of human remains crashing through the window of the pub. My father was off duty at the time from Commando training and was visiting my mother since they were engaged. So, I know all too well the imprinted effect this and countless other trauma-related imprints had on my parents and grandparents.

As a child in Manchester, England, I lived through the daily power cuts of 1973. This was when the union strikes severely restricted coal mining for power stations, combined with oil restrictions due to the embargo, and overall massive inflation caused the country to be forced into only working a 3-day week. The government was therefore forced to conserve electricity, hence the daily rotating power cuts which regularly left us in the dark each evening. Thankfully, some of my parents wartime-like supplies came in quite handy in those days. I remember how each evening we would sit around a single candle in the living room. We had only burn one candle at a time simply because we had no idea how long the power cuts would last for and consequently candles were in short supply. The imprint this left on me that I have carried throughout my life was to always have more torches (flashlights) than I could ever use. This is because I was young, and the trauma of the crisis had been so deeply imprinted on my brain that it became a habit to always have a torch (flashlight) to hand for the rest of my life.

Today, loneliness is a very real danger for millions of people. This is not simply a feeling that will pass because for many they need external connections for their very survival. Unfortunately, because of the enforced pandemic lockdown, for millions across the globe, there are few, if any, ways to make those essential external connections.

Make no mistake, loneliness is a real killer. Loneliness and the cascade of after-effects it carries with it can induce obesity, heart disease, clinical depression, depressed hormone levels, low self-esteem, feelings of guilt, feelings of worthlessness, feelings of despair, feelings of guilt, and even suicide. The fact is the human beings need to connect with others, it is a biological imperative.

A Little Can Mean a Lot

At this time when so many are acutely suffering the feelings of loneliness and anxiety, a little can mean a lot. Even while observing strict pandemic social distancing restrictions everyone can help those in need with a little forethought and effort.

For example, in the area where we live there is an old man who repeatedly walks up and down the Wilmslow Road multiple every day, all day. From around 0600hrs, rain or shine, winter, or summer until about 2100hrs, John (not his real name) walks between Great Western Street and Didsbury Village, which can be easily searched online. This is a one-way distance of 4.5 miles and at an average walking speed it takes about 1 hour and 30 minutes for a 9-mile, 3-hour round trip. I have calculated that if he does this trip 6 times each day, he covers 27 miles; and we have never once seen anyone stop and talk with him to simply say hello.

Since my wife and I walk with our dog on a similar albeit shorter route 4 times a day, we make it a priority to time our walks when we believe we will have the best chance of running into him so we can say hello and have a chat. Over the years we learned his name, we learned that his lodgings require him to be out from 6 am and he can only return at 9 am. We learned that he rarely, if ever, has anyone stop and say hello to him. We have given money even though he has never asked for it, we have made and also bought sandwiches and drinks, we have bought him clothes, and have invited him to join us for dinner.

Now, as a result of the pandemic lockdown, the streets are like those of a ghost town. Even at a peak period, there is hardly a soul to be seen. We also know that this will make him feel even more isolated and uncared for than ever. Therefore, even though we cannot do very much in real terms, we maintain our timing so that we stand the best chances of rendezvousing with John at some point. We cannot stand and chat as we used to do, but we can still make a point of standing at a distance, sometimes over the road, while we catch up and listen to the stories he loves to share. It is almost like in recanting the stories of his younger years they become a happy place for him to be in that moment. We also make a point of arranging to meet up roughly at the same place at the same times during each day, and also every day. We feel this may be another anchor point of contact and human interaction which may make a huge difference to him. We sincerely wish that we could do more, and we will try in the future if we see an opportunity to help.

What we do is not very much. It costs little or nothing except a tiny bit of time and effort, and yet it makes him smile and laugh a few times each day. It makes a difference. Things like writing a note for a neighbour who lives alone, send a text, offer to go shopping, make a phone call, and wave or say hello (at an appropriate distance) to someone you may not know but whom you see each day etc. If you do strike up a conversation with a person you know lives alone and/or has few or no friends, then keep your conversations on the positive side. Also, encourage them not to watch or listen to the barrage of mainstream media who love to make a drama out of any situation just for the sake of an attention-grabbing headline. In short, a little can mean a lot, and everyone can help.

We cannot solve the problem of millions of people around the world suffering loneliness and enable them to somehow be able to connect with others at the level they need to maintain good mental health.

However, we can help everyone who feels the effects of loneliness and despair to feel a little better in just 70 seconds. This is not a great panacea. However, it is a positive step on the pathway to creating some semblance of stability and promote a feel-good factor each day. Something to look forward to, and something that will have a positive cascade effect that pays dividends throughout each isolation day in many other ways.

A Broken Heart Can Kill You

Research is now strongly suggesting that emotional stress can physically kill you. This means that everyone who suffers loneliness, anxiety, and depression etc., are at risk to some degree.

An excellent, albeit an incredibly sad example of how emotional stress can be a killer, occurred when Star Wars actress Carrie Fisher died on December the 27th 2016. Her mother was actress Debbie Reynolds and was quoted as saying that "I miss her so much I just want to be with her." Hours later, Debbie Reynolds died too.

Debbie Reynolds could have fallen victim to what is known as Takotsubo Cardiomyopathy, AKA *Broken Heart Syndrome*. The consultant cardiologist at Birmingham City Hospital, Dr Derek Connolly was quoted in the media at the time as suggesting this.

It seems that Takotsubo Cardiomyopathy usually happens in the 48-hour window after someone suffers a bereavement. Also, since the symptoms are shortness of breath, and chest and arm pain etc., it is challenging for doctors to differentiate between a heart attack and Takotsubo Cardiomyopathy. The science suggests that the body suffers because the stress triggers the release of massive quantities of hormones like adrenalin which in squeezing the heart muscles can starve them of blood.

The effect that our mental health can have on our physical bodies is now well documented. Our mental health can have a direct and powerful impact on us in many different ways. For example, research suggests that within 12 months of losing a spouse the surviving partner is up to 67% more likely to suffer a heart attack. This is a frightening, yet extremely powerful example of how our mental health can physically kill us without us doing anything to make that happen except thinking about it and wishing it.

Anxiety

What is the difference between anxiety and depression? This is a particularly good question and I will briefly summarise the key differences. Typically, anxiety is not triggered by a single factor. Instead, it usually comes as a reaction to a combination of factors such as work-related matters, exams, debt, and physical health issues etc. However, the anxiety experienced by those suffering from an anxiety condition is different. This is because it is not necessarily connected with the aforementioned external factors and the anxiety is persistent and ever-present which has a direct impact on life quality and how we function daily. The common signs and symptoms include the following.

- Racing pulse
- Rapid breathing pattern
- Shortness of breath
- Irritability
- Panic attacks
- Feeling extreme fear
- Deliberately avoiding people, places, events, and things that you associate with feeling anxious

Depression

We can all feel down, sad, low, and moody from time to time, this is just all part of life and how we deal with things we encounter along the way. Typically, these feelings of being in a slump are usually caused by some specific reason or reasons which will change and pass.

Therefore, for most of us, these feelings thankfully do not usually last too long and we metaphorically pick ourselves up, brush ourselves off, our inner monologue says something like, "Come on, pull yourself together" and we then deal with the issues at hand and get on with life as our mood lifts.

However, for some, these feelings can last for weeks, months or even years for no apparent reason. Therefore, you may be depressed if you suffer like this for long periods and have experienced more than one symptom simultaneously. This is when you should seek professional help and consult your doctor immediately.

Mental Health and Exercise

There is an old axiom which is, a healthy body means a healthy mind. In general, this is true. It is also equally true in reverse, in that a healthy mind means a healthy body. Without a doubt, regular exercise and our overall wellbeing are inextricably linked.

One research study found that we are up to 25% less likely to develop depression and or anxiety issues if we follow a regular exercise regimen. Also, regular exercise has been proven to combat overall fatigue, it makes us more alert and better able to function cognitively and gives us improved focus and concentration.

Some studies have strongly suggested that something as simple as a 10-minute walk can be the equal of an hour-long exercise class or time in a gym. This makes something as simple as walking an important, easy to perform, and inexpensive exercise tool when it comes to combatting stress and depression.

Interestingly, concerning generating the feel-good experience through exercise, it is not all about the volume of exercise performed that makes the key difference. This is a good thing because if you are feeling low or depressed, it is not always easy to generate the enthusiasm to take a walk, let alone perform a lengthy exercise routine or class.

It seems that the key to generating the feel-good experience through exercise can be all about the intensity of exercise that is performed. More importantly, it does not have to be exceptionally high-intensity exercise that is needed. This means that the easily achievable target 2/3rds (66.67%) of a person's overall maximum intensity needed for the 10-exercise total-body isometric exercise workout routine of The 70 Second Difference™ can make all the difference to mental health.

Naturally, the beneficial effect of exercise does not last long, so regular exercise is needed to sustain the beneficial effect. We do not see this as a drawback because even though we may have enjoyed our last meal at dinner last evening, the effect soon wears off and we need to eat again before too long. We believe that this is how we should treat taking regular exercise. It should be something that we just do every day as naturally as eating and drinking.

Depression, Mood and Exercise

It is now well known and documented that exercise and be an effective treatment for depression. Exercise has far fewer side-effects than medication, which is a huge benefit in itself. Also, there is no stigma attached to taking regular exercise as opposed to taking anti-depressants and undergoing regular counselling sessions.

Exercise will lift your mood and make you feel more positive as a result. Many other positive feelings come as a result of taking an exercise session, and it is interesting to note that some studies suggest that exercise can be most beneficial when we feel particularly low.

Exercise is now also increasingly recognised as being beneficial in combatting dementia. Studies suggest that regular exercise reduces the likelihood of general cognitive decline and for those who already have dementia, exercise can significantly delay functional decline.

In relation to exercise and mood, one of the first things people think about is endorphins. Endorphins are technically neurotransmitters produced in the pituitary gland in response to stress which allow the transmission of electrical signals from one neuron to another via synapses. Endorphins are endogenous which means that they originate from within the body.

Endorphins make us feel good because they interact with the opiate receptors in the brain. In doing so, they reduce the perception of pain in a similar way to morphine etc. Since endorphins are produced in response to pain and stress, this is why the physical discomfort and stress of exercise produces them. This is because the body cannot differentiate between harmful pain and injury and beneficial intense exercise. During intense exercise, our body increases the production of neurotransmitters such as serotonin and norepinephrine, and the same mechanism that triggers the production of endorphins also triggers the production of endocannabinoids such as anandamide which creates a calming feeling. In short, the body produces a form of internal cannabis through exercise.

The mind-body link can no longer be ignored, and exercise should be promoted and used to not only make us physically fitter and healthier but also for our mental health too. Our overall wellbeing is all-encompassing in the mind-body link.

The 70 Second Difference™

The 70 Second Difference™ is a protocol based upon the premise that 70 seconds of consecutive exercise time is the time needed to perform a 10-exercise total-body workout routine using the scientifically proven isometric exercise system.

Research has shown that physical exercise can help you to combat depression, bolster your self-worth, make you fitter and stronger, and simply make you feel better in general.

One of the drawbacks to exercise is that not everyone enjoys it, not everyone wants to spend long doing it, and not everyone has the equipment needed to exercise with. Also, especially during self-isolation at home, there is not the option of simply going to the gym to have a workout. Besides, not everyone has the money to spend in joining a gym or buying expensive home exercise equipment.

This is where The 70 Second Difference™ makes a huge difference. This is because you do not need any special exercise equipment, you do not need a coach or any special knowledge because the exercises are some of the simplest imaginable, almost anyone can perform them, and you do not need lots so space because if you can stand up and sit down then you have a total-body workout. The best part is that they are scientifically proven to work.

To follow The 70 Second Difference™ protocol all you need to do is to perform 10 simple exercises each day. Each exercise lasts for just 7 seconds, hence why we call it The 70 Second Difference™. That is, it, nothing more is needed. The results will be that you will begin to feel just a little better after your very first workout. The results you get will build up little by little, layer by layer, day by day and in exchange for just 70 seconds of consecutive exercise time each day.

As you push during an exercise imagine pushing away any depression you might feel, as you pull during an exercise imagine pulling only good feelings back to you, and as you lift during an exercise imagine lifting your mood and feeling better.

Even if you are someone who has never exercised before, provided you are in good health and have a medical clearance to exercise from your doctor, then just 70 seconds of consecutive exercise time can make all the difference. It can make the difference between feeling sad or happy, between bad or good, between down or up, and between negative or positive.

Give it a go with an open mind and see for yourself the difference that The 70 Second Difference™ can make to how you feel. Before we get to the exercise section, we will explain a little more about the science behind it all and the background to the system etc. Please note that this book together with the science and exercise in it is a condensed form of many of the subjects that are in expanded from the book The 70 Second Difference™.

To close this section, I am going to quote one of the greatest motivational speakers of all time, Zig Ziglar. Zig was a mentor when I was a young man, and I am proud to say that he became a friend later in life. During his outstanding career, Zig has said many famous things which are now frequently quoted by motivational experts and psychologists. One for the things Zig is most famous for saying is "You are what you are because of what goes into your mind."

However, at this juncture, I will remember him by offering another of his perhaps more fitting quotes, "Logic will not change a feeling or emotion, only a physical action will." Of course, Zig is absolutely correct. This is why we urge you to change the way you feel with the physical action of The 70 Second Difference™ exercise protocol.

21 Days to a New Habit?

Over the years there has been a lot of discussion amongst motivational speakers, NLP experts (Neuro-Linguistic Programming) and psychologists about how to form new positive habits. It has often been boldly quoted that you can form a new habit in as little as 21 days, but is this true?

From my experience and research, I believe that a new habit takes root in as little as 21 days, but this is only the start. For many, the 21-day root planting exercise creates enough of an anchor point to allow them to build a new positive habit from that point onwards. However, for others, it may take a little longer.

This is good news for those who have never exercised regularly before, and yet want to form a new habit to perform a simple 10 x 7-second total-body exercise routine as per The 70 Second Difference™ protocol.

First, let us look at what a habit is. Habits are behaviours which we automatically perform simply because they have been performed so frequently. Performing something frequently eventually creates a mental association between an action and a behaviour. These are also commonly known as the cue and the behaviour. When we encounter a cue, a linked behaviour is then automatically performed without conscious thought about what we are doing. In other words, we do something out of habit.

What we need to do is to create a cue to make the behaviour of performing The 70 Second Difference™ exercise protocol every day become a habit. However, just because you can eventually form a new habit to exercise regularly it does not mean to say that your old habit of not exercising will disappear. Instead, you need to work on making the new habit stronger than the old one so that it takes priority.

A researcher from University College London, Dr Phillippa Lally, suggests that a new habit can take as long as 66 days to first form, and up to 254 days to fully form. Naturally, some people formed new habits very quickly, in 21 days or not much more, while others in the studies took longer. Also, research results will always vary because everyone is different. On average though, the time taken to form a new habit was much longer than many may wish you to believe, but facts must be faced in the wake of solid research. For those who wish to read the research report in full, the results were published in the European Journal of Social Psychology.

This is still good news because it still means that you can form a positive new habit, however, for some people, not all, it may take a little longer than it was first thought.

How do you create a new habit to perform The 70 Second Difference™ exercise protocol every day? You simply need to repeat the same procedure every day in the same situation. If you ensure that as many elements remain constant every day, then this will help tremendously. Try wearing the same clothes, exercising in the same place, facing in the same direction, and especially at the same time. If you like music, then play the same music every day while you exercise. The more cues/triggers you can create the better, and the faster the new exercise habit will form.

Set yourself up to succeed rather than fail. Little things can make a big difference, so plan out your day. Make sure that you avoid listening to the news because this is normally negative and even if it is on in the background your subconscious mind still absorbs the negativity. Try to ensure that everyone around you has some sort of positive association for you to help feed your mind the right way every day.

Take baby steps. Do not expect to go from a standing start to exercising at full force right away. Once you have learned how to perform the exercises and learned how to breathe correctly, then these will shift from your conscious mind into your subconscious. From there you can then begin to gradually apply a little more intensity into each exercise you perform. Remember, the more intensity you can safely apply, then the better the results that you will achieve. However, always exercise within your safe limits.

Consistency is always the key to success, and very soon you will find it becomes progressively easier for you to exercise each day. Once the process starts to shift how to exercise and breathe correctly into your subconscious mind then you are well on your way to developing the new habit you want and need.

Chapter 2: Exercise Science Overview

In this section, we will give a user-friendly overview of exercise science together with the features and benefits of various exercise techniques and concepts. For those who want more in-depth information about the science of isometric exercise and health and fitness in general, then we suggest that you also read our books The ISOmetric Bible™ and The 70 Second Difference™ books. Both are available on Amazon.

The Basic Types of Resistance Exercise

All muscle training falls into between two or three specific categories, depending upon how you break them down. In the most basic form, there are two types, either contraction with movement, or contraction without movement. Breaking them down a step further there become three categories, with one being isotonic, another isokinetic. Last but certainly not the least, is isometric.

Isotonic training is all about movement with muscle shortening and lengthening during the lifting and lowering phases of the exercise. We know that the isotonic category can be broken down further into three parts. One part being the concentric contraction, which is the lifting phase of an exercise when the muscles shorten in length. Another is the eccentric phase which is the lowering part of an exercise when the muscles lengthen.

Lastly in this isotonic category is the isokinetic contraction. This is where the muscle changes in length during both the concentric and eccentric phases of the contraction, however, the velocity remains constant no matter how much force is applied during the exercises.

Then comes the isometric category. With an isometric exercise, there is no movement whatsoever. To help you envision this in, I will take a random weight training or freehand callisthenic exercise such as a chest press because it can be performed either with movement OR without movement, as an isometric exercise.

For example, a barbell, a machine, or your bodyweight can be lifted and lowered to perform an exercise such as a barbell curl, this is called, isotonic exercise, callisthenics or simply exercise with movement.

To perform the same or similar exercise isometrically you would attempt to perform the same or similar biomechanically correct actions of a barbell curl, however, at a certain point, or points if multiple exercise points were being used, the curling movement would stop because an immovable object point had been reached.

At that point or points, you would apply an increasing level of intensity until you reach the desired target level as you attempt to perform the curling exercise against the immovable object.

At the desired isometric exercise point, a constant force is applied against the immovable object for 7 seconds which is the optimum isometric exercise time. The ideal basic isometric exercise point for general exercise is roughly at the mid-point when your muscles reach a stalemate working against each other or an immovable object. This is called a Standard isometric Contraction.

The harder you engage your muscles as you try to break the stalemate by lifting, pushing, or pulling, then the stronger your muscles become. In doing so, you engage many more muscle fibres than normal as you attempt to move the immovable object and perform the curling exercise action.

Doors, desks, chairs, walls, and many other everyday items work well as immovable objects BUT the easiest and most used immovable object is typically yourself.

Isometric Overview

As you now know, isometric exercise does not involve any movement. Instead, the joint angle and the muscle length do not change during contraction. You also now know that 7 seconds is now regarded as the optimum time to perform an isometric exercise.

However, almost everyone when exercising tends to count the exercise elapsed time much faster than real elapsed time. This means that it is easy not to reach the magic 7 seconds of the optimum isometric exercise time. Therefore, we always suggest aiming to perform the exercise for 10 seconds to ensure that the 7-second target is always reached even when under the stress of performing intense exercise.

Isometric exercise has been extensively scientifically researched and has been proven time and again to be a highly efficient way to build great strength and grow muscle. In fact, isometric exercise is probably one of the most thoroughly researched of all exercise systems.

However, it also remains one of the most misunderstood systems of exercises. This is almost certainly through fear, professional ignorance and for purely financial reasons.

Several different techniques can be used in the isometric exercise system. Most of these techniques are highly advanced for use by competitive athletes, competitive martial arts practitioners, strength athletes and bodybuilders. Therefore, they have no application as part of a general isometric exercise session for the average person who simply wants to get generally stronger and fitter.

However, purely out of interest I will list them here, and in case any fitness enthusiast, athletes or bodybuilders read this book and wish to try them. They are described in greater detail in our book called The Isometric Bible which is available on Amazon and good bookstores. The most common and advanced isometric exercise techniques include the following:

- Standard Isometric Contraction
- Yielding Isometric Contraction
- Maximum Duration Isometrics
- Oscillatory Isometrics
- Impact Absorption Isometrics
- Explosive Isometrics, AKA: Ballistic Isometrics
- Static-Dynamic Isometric
- Isometric Contrast
- Functional Isometrics
- TRISOmetrics™

There are more than enough isometric exercises that can be performed without any equipment whatsoever to allow a total body workout routine to be completed relatively easily. These will typically be self-resisted isometric exercises, which are excellent. However, by using only minimal readily available equipment such as walking poles, golf clubs, martial arts belts, climbing ropes, scuba diving webbing weight belts, and broom handles etc. it is possible to greatly expand the number of exercises that can be performed.

It is also perfectly possible to adapt and use other readily available items such as tow ropes, steel chains, towels, and commonly found immobile objects such as sturdy fixed barrier railings, solid walls, solid doors, door frames, or parked vehicles to perform a complete isometric exercise routine. Again, these are all excellent improvised exercise tools which allow an expanded range of highly effective isometric exercises to be performed.

Using improvised exercise tools can yield an unexpected additional benefit. This is that it allows one to focus more and apply greater concentration to each exercise. This is particularly useful for those who are either completely new to, or who are relatively new to the isometric exercise system. We will explain more about what these can be later in the book.

One of the things we love about both the isometric and self-resisted system of exercise is that as you get stronger through exercise, then you can apply more force and intensity to your isometric or self-resisted exercises.

This, in turn, means that you can gradually increase the level of intensity you can safely apply to each exercise which will mean that the results and benefits you receive will grow in a compound way through regular daily use. This is what we call a natural Adaptive Response™ mechanism which is a useful aspect of our biology.

Isometric Exercise Science

Even until the mid-20th century, there was almost no scientific research that had been performed into the benefits of isometric exercise. We also know that before the first serious scientific research study, how people trained isometrically was typically by performing what we now call endurance isometrics.

Thankfully, isometric exercise has now been thoroughly scientifically researched and proven for several decades. I would estimate that there has probably been at least as much scientific research performed into isometric exercise as there has into traditional resistance training.

The first major in-depth study into isometric exercise was performed at the world-famous Max Plank Institute in Dortmund, Germany. If you already have a reasonable knowledge of science, you will also know that the Max Plank Institute is a world-renowned centre of scientific excellence in many disciplines. Between 1953 and 1958, one of the most extensive research studies was commissioned into isometric exercise science. These experiments are now considered by many to be the original "gold standard" of all isometric exercise studies. It was first made public knowledge in the resultant ground-breaking book, "The Physiology of Strength," by Dr Theodor Hettinger - Research Fellow at the Max Plank Institute.

During that 5-year research period, Dr Hettinger and Dr Muller perform over 5,500 experiments on volunteers from all walks of life, and at every level of strength, fitness, and athletic ability. The test subjects even included serious strength athletes and middle-aged, overweight, and unfit people of both sexes.

Perhaps what surprised people the most was how dramatic and impressive the results which were gained from performing isometric exercises. Also, because the same or similar results were easily repeatable it made the data gained from the experiments exceptionally reliable.

The conclusion of the extensive studies proved beyond doubt the overall superiority of isometric exercise when it comes to building both strength and muscle, compared to traditional isotonic exercises methods. It also proved that the isometric system delivered these results much faster and with far less exercise than through traditional resistance training.

Another extremely interesting result emerged from the experiments. This was that it was not the length of time that an isometric exercise was held that produced the optimum results. Instead, it was the correct level of intensity applied for a very specific optimum time.

They found that by performing only one daily isometric exercise for between only 6 and 7 seconds, and at only two-thirds of an individual's maximum effort, it could increase strength by an average of up to 5% per week. By any standards, strength gains of 5% in exchange for the expenditure of only 66%, or around two-thirds of an individual's maximum capacity, is an excellent result.

Perhaps even more amazingly, they discovered that after someone has performed a single 7-second training stimulus (exercise) per day, the muscle being exercised in that same position was no longer responsive to further gains. In other words, it did not matter how many more times you exercised the same muscle in the same position, there would be no further increase in muscle growth or strength. The only way to do this was to perform another isometric exercise at a different position only the ROM (Range Of Motion) of the limb being exercised. The scientific data about this can be referenced on pages 28 to 31 of Dr Theodor Hettinger's book, "The Physiology of Strength."

In 2001, Nicolas Babault PhD of the University of Burgundy, Dijon, France, led a team of scientists to research and examine how many muscle fibres were activated, and how long they remained active for, during both traditional weight training and in isometric training.

(*The scientific research paper is published: Nicolas Babault, Michel Pousson, Yves Ballay, and Jacques Van Hoecke - Groupe Analyse du Mouvement, Unite´ de Formation et de Recherche Sciences et Techniques des Activite´s Physiques et Sportives, Universite´ de Bourgogne, BP 27877, 21078 Dijon Cedex, France.*)

They discovered that when training intensely, and in near-perfect style, the levels of muscle activation during repetitions of optimum maximal weight training were between 89.7% during the concentric contraction, or when lifting a weight, and 88.3% during the eccentric contraction, or when lowering a weight. For practical purposes, an average of about 89% overall.

The study also revealed that during the lifting, or concentric part of the exercise, the maximum intramuscular tension only lasted for between 0.25 and 0.5 seconds. Which, for practical purposes is an average of about 1/3rd of a second during each isotonic repetition.

This is because traditional isotonic resistance exercises naturally involve movement. They also have aspects of velocity and acceleration to consider in the overall equation. "Force" is only produced for a split second, to produce a maximal contraction of the muscle fibres.

The same research also showed that the level of muscle activation during isometric exercise was as high as 95.2% and that it lasted for the entire 7 to 10 seconds of each exercise. This is a huge increase over the 1/3rd of second muscular activation achieved during a single repetition of weight training.

Therefore, based on these discoveries, then technically a single isometric exercise performed at only two-thirds of an individual's overall maximum can deliver either similar or often even better results, than the equivalent of up to 3 sets of 10 weight training repetitions in the lifting phase of the exercise.

To explain this further I will use a typical barbell curl exercise in the lifting phase as my example, where the object of the exercise is to engage as many muscle fibres as possible in a maximum muscular contraction. Naturally, 3 sets of 10 repetitions give us an overall total of 30 repetitions. One set of 10 repetitions of the barbell curl in perfect high-intensity style produces a total maximum muscular engagement for a total of approximately 3.3 seconds. Three sets of 10 repetitions of the same exercise, a total of 30 repetitions, this will give a total of approximately 9.9 seconds of maximum muscular engagement, and an average of 89% muscle activation overall.

In comparison, if one high-intensity isometric contraction exercise produces a maximum muscular engagement that lasts for the entire duration of the exercise. Even though the optimum time over which an isometric exercise is performed was found to be 7 seconds, this is almost always rounded up to the 10-second target number. The maximum muscular engagement will last for the entire 10 seconds of a high-intensity isometric exercise and with 95.2% muscle activation overall.

This is proof that is based entirely on scientific research that 3 sets of 10 near-perfect high-intensity curls when weight training, which takes several minutes to perform, still was not equal to the results achieved by a single 10-second high-intensity isometric curl exercise.

The Standard Isometric Contraction

The standard isometric contraction is a simple and highly effective technique. Therefore, this is the technique we will focus on for practical isometric training.

The standard isometric contraction, AKA: overcoming isometric contraction, AKA: maximum-effort isometrics, or whatever else you wish to call it, is when a muscle is applying force to push or pull against an immovable resistance. This is the most basic of all kinds of isometric exercise, and it is highly effective.

This type of isometric contraction exercise was performed during the experiments by Dr T. Hettinger and Dr E. Muller at the Max Plank Institute. It is also the technique referred to in their book "The Physiology of Strength".

In a standard isometric contraction, it is theoretically possible to exert up to 100% of one's maximum capacity effort against an immovable object and then continue to hold that level of intensity throughout the exercise. This means that standard isometric contraction can be a very high-intensity exercise system.

In performing an isometric exercise against an immovable object at a certain level of intensity for a given duration of time it will teach your body to recruit more muscle fibres to try to move the object. As you perform the exercise and generate as much force as possible, your CNS, or Central Nervous System, learns that it needs to activate and recruit more muscle fibres to reach the goal of moving the object.

Since this will naturally be impossible to move, the process will continue each time you exercise to make you stronger and grow more muscle. Your body mechanisms become trained to readily activate and recruit additional muscle fibres as needed when facing repeated similar challenges, which in turn, repeats the cycle more readily every time.

As we mentioned earlier, the immovable/solid object that is used can be anything that is completely solid and completely safe to use. This can be a wall, a door, door jamb, parked motor vehicle or anything similar. Perhaps the most common objects used to enhance everyday isometric exercise training are sturdy towels, climbing rope, martial arts belts, scuba diving weight belts, webbing straps, golf clubs, and broom handles, etc. All the aforementioned items are excellent when used properly, and all will deliver some excellent results. More importantly, they are typically readily available for most people which makes exercising with them so much easier.

Another common way to perform isometric exercise is to do it in a self-resisted way. Self-resisted means that you push or pull against your limbs, hands, and feet, etc. For example, you might place the palms of your hands together at chest level with your hands roughly at the midpoint of your body. In that position, you would then press your hands together using your chest muscles to provide the primary driving force. Suddenly, you are performing a highly effective self-resisted isometric chest exercise!

It is possible to perform a well-balanced and highly effective self-resisted isometric workout to exercise virtually every section of the body. So, never underestimate self-resisted exercise because it can be immensely powerful indeed. Also, self-resistance exercises are an excellent way to ensure that a personal maximum resistance is used safely, and with minimum risk of injury caused by applying too much force.

The fact is that it does not matter which method is chosen. It can be isometrics performed against an immovable object, self-resisted isometrics, or a combination of the two. The most important thing is that either the object must be completely immovable through human muscle power alone, or the force of one body-part must be able to completely counterbalance the force of another body-part to produce a muscular stalemate.

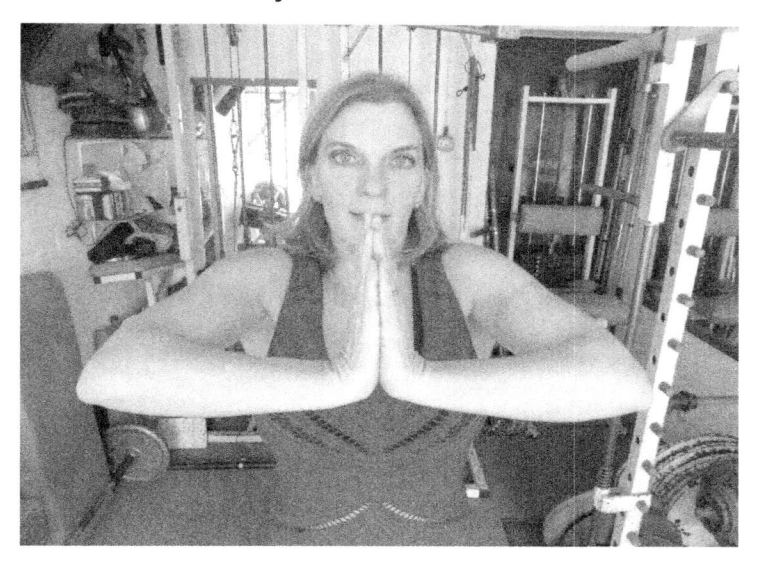

Workout Intensity

Intensity is always going to be a relative term, and it is often completely misunderstood when it is used concerning exercise. When it comes to exercising your muscles, the intensity is the % of your ability to move a resistance. Technically, an individual's highest possible level of intensity is when they reach a point of momentary failure after exerting themselves completely.

However, the important questions we need to try and find answers to are: "How hard is hard?" and "How intense is intense?" To some degree, both are very subjective things. Taking two people of roughly equal fitness, something that is intense to one person might be considered comparatively easy to the other.

Hard is a relative term, and handling 50 lbs of resistance is impossibly hard if your strength is only at the level required to lift 49 lbs. However, if you can lift a 100 lbs as a maximum, then lifting 50 lbs is going to be comparatively easy.

Often, the only factors differentiating between people and the intensity level exerted, are going to be mental toughness, determination, and perception.

Therefore, to gain the greatest benefits from isometric exercise the first thing that must be learned is how to determine, with a reasonable degree of accuracy, what level of intensity is being applied to an exercise.

It is just a fact that what one person deems to be 100% of their capacity will always be quite different from another person's estimate. The accurate estimation of what one person deems to be $2/3^{rds}$ of their overall maximum intensity will also vary from person to person. The accuracy of estimation will also vary greatly between an experienced professional athlete and an absolute beginner to exercise.

Experience has taught us that most people who are new to exercise will always fall well short of accurate estimation of any given percentage. A beginner will find it more challenging to accurately estimate what $2/3^{rds}$ of their 100% maximum is when compared to a more experienced athlete. Many people might believe that they are performing at 100% capacity when they are only performing at around only 2/3rds, or even perhaps at only 50% or less of their 100% maximum.

This is because exercise is new to them, therefore, the experiences and feelings in their body which are associated with it are also new. They simply have no common frame of reference when it comes to calculating/estimating their level of physical exertion.

The human brain has a built-in mechanism which helps to protect the body and prevent it from performing physical activity to such a level that could cause serious damage or even death. This is the mechanism that makes your brain tell you to stop exercising when it begins to get tough, and the feeling of wanting to stop exercising only increases as you continue to push yourself harder to do more. This is all despite the biological fact that you are physically capable of doing much more than is being suggested by the messages you are receiving from yourself.

Over time, the brain of people who exercise regularly, and especially to a high level of intensity, will naturally adjust, and reposition this built-in safety margin. This means that the brain of an experienced high-level athlete does not "tell" them to stop an exercise until the level of intensity is much higher than it would be for a beginner.

Therefore, when it comes to exercise, how is it possible to subjectively quantify, and then impart appropriate levels of recommended intensity? This problem is made even more challenging when one considers the fact that accurately translating and subjectively assessing various levels of intensity will, to some degree, always be subjective to every individual.

If you were to train as hard as humanly possible, with near 100% maximum intensity which involves super-strict form, and training to complete failure and beyond, then you simply cannot train for a long time. It is just physiologically impossible. Physics and biology are quite simple in this respect.

The intensity of your workout is directly proportional to the length of time that you are physically able to perform your workout. The harder and more intensely you exercise, then the shorter time that you will be physically able to perform the exercise.

Make no mistake, performing a 7-second isometric exercise while exerting close to your personal 100% maximum physical capacity is completely and utterly exhausting, even for a professional athlete.

What does all this mean when it comes to accurately communicate various levels of exercise intensity, especially when there is no professional coach or elaborate and expensive measuring equipment at hand?

Research clearly shows that almost everyone will stop exercising long before they are in any danger of becoming seriously fatigued. Most people will *think* they are achieving a much higher level of intensity than they would do if they were only a little more mentally resilient.

This does not mean that people should suddenly begin pushing themselves beyond their physical limits, which would be a stupid thing to do. However, it does mean that most people who enjoy a higher than average level of mental resilience and determination, as well as being in physically good condition, can push themselves much harder than they might think. If anyone ever feels "genuine" strain or fatigue to the point of becoming injured, then they should stop exercising immediately.

Even without the aid of a professional coach to monitor, encourage you and measure your intensity and progress with specialist equipment, the tips we have outlined in this section will help you to get the most out every workout. It is also worth remembering that if you cheat, then the only person who loses is "you."

Technically, How Does a Muscle Grow?

How does a muscle grow? This is one of the most common questions asked concerning fitness and exercise in general. However, it is also one of the most misunderstood concepts, even amongst fitness professionals and personal trainers. To see for yourself just how uninformed or badly informed some people are, simply join one or two of the social media groups online so you can read some of the absolute drivel posted by 'keyboard warriors' who purport to be 'experts' on the subject. Alarmingly, many of these people seem to have developed a hardcore following, which to the science-based professional is like watching 'fools leading other fools' on a wild goose chase.

So, back to the key question which is, how does a muscle grow? To explain this, we must examine three concepts, which are: 1) muscle growth through increases in the volume/size of myofibrils inside the muscles, which is commonly termed as being myofibrillar hypertrophy. 2) hyperplasia, which is when there is an increase in the number of muscle cells/fibres. 3) sarcoplasmic growth which is all about increasing the fluid content.

When it comes to the subject of exercise, the muscles you wish to grow must be challenged with a workload which is greater than they can currently accommodate. In other words, exercise that is intense enough to stimulate growth. This stimulus can come from any source such as lifting a heavy object, weight training, isometrics, through compressing a spring in a device such as a Bullworker™, or through self-resistance either hand to hand / limb to limb / using an Iso-Bow™ etc.

This process creates trauma to the muscle fibres which disrupts the muscle cell organelles. This then triggers other cells outside the muscle fibres to greatly increase in numbers at and around the point of the trauma to repair the damage. The process of repair involves a fusion of cells. This, in turn, causes the cross-sectional area of the muscle fibre to increase because the muscle cell myofibrils increase in both size and quantity. This process is more commonly known as hypertrophy. Since this process increases the number of cellular nuclei the muscle fibres generate more myosin and actin. These are contractile protein myofilaments which in turn help to make the muscle stronger.

To summarize, this is the basis of what is more commonly known as myofibril muscle growth. In addition to this, there is also probably a process called hyperplasia which takes place. I use the term, 'probably' because this concept is extremely controversial for many reasons. One of the key problems being that evidence of this in human beings is lacking, whereas there is a mass of evidence supporting hyperplasia in mice and other animals.

Hypertrophy is the increase in the size of the existing muscle fibres to accommodate the increased demands placed upon them through intense exercise. Hyperplasia, concerning skeletal muscle growth, is the increase in the number of muscle fibres which in turn will also increase the cross-sectional area of a muscle.

Despite there being a lack of evidence supporting hyperplasia in human beings, logic supports the process taking place. This is because of a theory known as Nuclear Domain Theory. This states that the nucleus of a cell (a muscle cell in this instance) is only able to control a finite area of cellular space. It is thought that satellite cells donate their nuclei to the muscle cell until a certain point is reached whereby this can no longer take place. Beyond a certain limit, and through continued intense training, the cell must eventually divide to create two cells instead of the former single cell. When this happens, the entire hypertrophy process starts over once again. This probably means that most of the muscle growth is almost certainly caused through hypertrophy, and a much smaller percentage can be attributed to hyperplasia at any given point in the muscle stimulus/growth process.

Finally, there is a subject of sarcoplasmic muscle growth to address. Sarcoplasmic muscle growth is the increase in the volume of sarcoplasmic fluid in the muscle cell. This is the fluid and energy resources surrounding the myofibrils in your muscles containing mostly glycogen together with other elements including creatine, ATP, and water etc.

To clarify, glycogen is simply a type of sugar that serves as a form of energy. It is deposited in bodily tissues as a store of carbohydrates, and it is the body's main form of storage for the sugar, glucose. Glycogen is stored in two main places in the body, one being the liver, and the other being the muscles.

More importantly, glycogen is the body's secondary source of long-term energy storage, with the primary energy storage source being fat. When glycogen is in the muscles, it is converted into glucose for use as energy when performing sports etc., and glycogen stored in the liver is converted into glucose for use as energy throughout the body, and in the central nervous system.

Therefore, sarcoplasmic growth increases the muscle volume, but this increase is not in functional strength mass since it does not increase the number of muscle fibres. It is like 'the pump', in that it is an increase in the size and shape of the muscle through the muscle holding an increased amount of fluid.

Rest Time Between Exercises

Naturally, the rest time taken between exercises during a workout is quite different from the rest and recovery needed to recover and allow your body to positively respond to the stimulus generated by exercise.

If you keep the rest time between exercises brief enough, then the workout routine itself will give you an excellent cardiovascular workout, and this is what we recommend that you ultimately aim for. If you are already very fit, then we would recommend that instead of performing the optional cardio routine, and you simply put more effort and intensity into each isometric exercise. At the same time, aim to keep the rest time between those exercises as brief as possible. This approach will help you work towards being able to perform each exercise so that it has an Ultra-High Intensity Ultra-Short Burst™ effect, which will greatly improve your overall fitness level, and boost your Base Metabolic Rate or BMR.

However, if you are not already fit, then to begin with you may wish to simply allow each isometric exercise to deliver all the cardio you need as you gradually build up your levels of fitness and endurance. Eventually, you will soon increase your level of fitness to a point where you can begin to gradually reduce the rest time between each exercise to a minimum point that works best for you.

Once you have learned how to fully engage the muscles during each exercise with sufficient intensity, and at the same time you have learned how to breathe fully, deeply, and naturally throughout each exercise. At the same time, you should be keeping the rest time between exercises to a minimum because this combination will have an excellent and beneficial cardiovascular effect.

Dynamic Flexation™

Dynamic Flexation™ is a technique we devised to help ensure that we gained maximum benefit from the isometric portion of our exercise regimens. I will recap and briefly summarise the Dynamic Flexation™ technique as originally laid out in "The 70 Second Difference™" book.

We always recommend that everyone who performs any kind of resistance exercise practices some form of Dynamic Flexation™ before performing any exercise. This will help to ensure that all muscles, tendons, ligaments, joints, and your spine have become naturally and properly engaged in the correct biomechanical exercise position.

We would never recommend that as soon as you assume any exercise position that you suddenly apply maximum power and intensity right away. This is unless you are a very experienced athlete, or unless you are training with a qualified coach to perform a certain type of isometric exercise to develop extra power such as a static-dynamic or explosive/ballistic isometric technique. Instead, we recommend that you always breathe naturally as you gradually flex and engage your muscles and joints into the exercise.

To perform Dynamic Flexation™ you gradually flex your grip and the muscles you are about to exercise while applying an increasing level of intensity immediately before performing the exercise. The exercised is then performed, and to disengage from the exercise we recommend reversing the Dynamic Flexation™ engagement process.

Our preference is to apply tension and intensity to the exercise gradually through Dynamic Flexation™ typically for between 2 and 3 seconds, or even for as long as 4 seconds if needed. This all takes place before beginning to count the required 7-second exercise time of the isometric contraction.

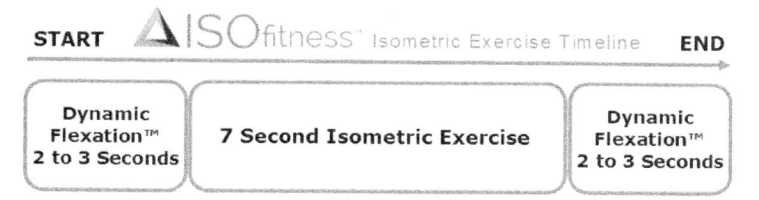

START △ISOfitness™ Isometric Exercise Timeline **END**

| Dynamic Flexation™ 2 to 3 Seconds | 7 Second Isometric Exercise | Dynamic Flexation™ 2 to 3 Seconds |

We prefer using one deep full breath in and out as a method of more accurately counting each second that has elapsed. This way, you will time each exercise more accurately, and you will not be tempted to hold your breath at any point which is a mistake that beginners often make.

Similarly, at the end of an exercise, we do not recommend that it be ended abruptly. Instead, we recommend reversing the Dynamic Flexation™ technique so that you gradually relax as you slightly move each muscle and joint out of the exercise position.

This process helps enormously because when you are in a good position it will help you to gain the maximum benefit from each exercise you perform. Dynamic Flexation™ is when you move and adjust either your feet, legs/leg, hips and especially your hands as you gradually assume a solid position and handgrip. As you flex and move, you will be making micro-adjustments.

All exercises will be performed best if you assume a correct and solid handgrip, fist clench, or foot position etc. One of the most important aspects of assuming the correct exercise position begins with your grip. Without a solid grip on a bar, handle, or anything else you need to hold while exercising, you will naturally be setting yourself up to perform sub-maximally. You can also be helping to develop injuries which can include sore elbows, joints, ligaments, and tendons.

Dynamic Flexation™ is a concept which embraces the broader principles of motor unit recruitment, and "Henneman's Size Principle" to increase the contractile strength of a muscle. Elwood Henneman's principle stated that under load, the motor units in a muscle are engaged according to their magnitude of force output, from the smallest to the largest, and in task-appropriate order.

This means that the slow-twitch, low-force, fatigue-resistant muscle fibres are activated before any fast-twitch, high-force muscle fibres are engaged which are less fatigue-resistant. Since the body naturally works in this way, it enables precise and finely controlled force to be delivered at all levels of output.

This also means that when exercising, or when performing tasks in daily life, the fatigue which is experienced as a result will be always be minimised. It will also be proportional to the sequential engagement of the most appropriate muscle fibres being engaged.

Isometric Exercises and Blood Pressure

Some exercise critics point out the fact that when someone performs an isometric exercise it will raise their blood pressure. However, the same people also very conveniently forget that the same is also true of all other forms of exercise including freehand callisthenics and traditional isotonic resistance training with weights.

ALL physical activity, and especially exercise will cause your blood pressure to rise for a short time. Providing that you are in good health, that you always breathe deeply, naturally, and normally when performing any exercise, then any rise in blood pressure will soon return to a normal level when the exercise is stopped. The faster this happens, the fitter you are.

For those who are advanced athletes and/or are used to hard and intense isometric training for a long time, then you will already have made significant progress in strengthening your heart and circulatory system.

For those who are new to isometric training, just like with any form of exercise, the best way into it is by taking it slowly and less intensely at first.

Newcomers to exercise, and especially isometrics, should always focus on applying less intensity, to begin with, and on always breathing fully and deeply throughout all exercises. NEVER HOLD YOUR BREATH!

Under strict medical supervision, even those with Coronary Artery Disease and high blood pressure should be able to increase their physical activity levels with a reasonable degree of safety safely. However, if you are a person who already suffers from high blood pressure, then you should always exercise at a much lower level of intensity than someone who has no physical issues.

Furthermore, **EVERYONE, AND ESPECIALLY PEOPLE WITH HYPERTENSION, OR ANY FORM OF CARDIOVASCULAR DISEASE, SHOULD ALWAYS CHECK WITH THEIR DOCTOR BEFORE BEGINNING ANY KIND OF EXERCISE ROUTINE.**

Rest and Recovery

When calculating your ideal recovery period, many things must be taking into consideration. These include your age, your current health and fitness level, the quantity of exercise taken, and most importantly the intensity of the exercise which has been performed.

Some people will need a recovery period of between 24 and 48 hours, and for others, the recovery period may be as brief as between 12 and 24 hours.

As a rule, the recovery period will always incrementally increase as the intensity of the exercises increases towards an individual's 100% potential maximum capacity. Always be aware of this and make sure that you factor this into your rest and recovery time calculations. The diagram will help to outline this.

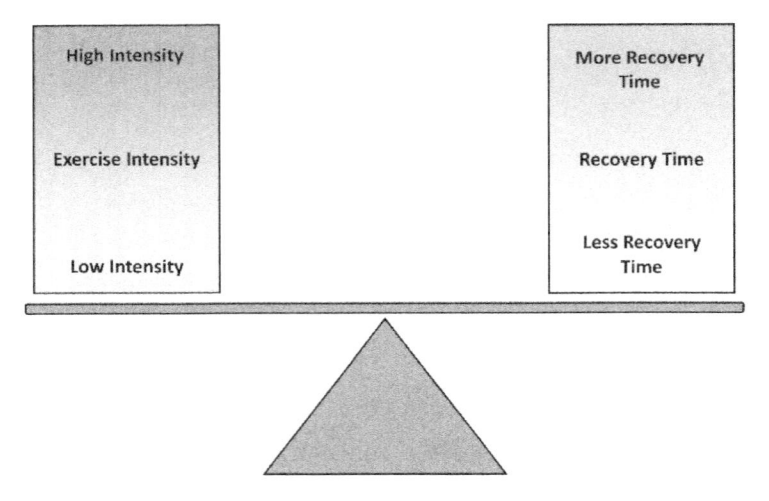

High Intensity		More Recovery Time
Exercise Intensity		Recovery Time
Low Intensity		Less Recovery Time

Sports scientist J. Atha's research revealed something remarkable. This was that when performing isometric contraction exercises at two-thirds of an individual's maximum capacity, the average person could safely perform an exercise like this daily, without overtraining.

Standard isometric contraction exercises can be safely performed daily, by almost anyone, of almost any age, and in almost any physical condition as a means of strength development, body shaping, and even for bodybuilding.

However, for more intense workouts, then we recommend a full rest day between workouts due to the higher demands being placed upon the Central Nervous System (CNS) and the time needed to fully recover and benefit from the exercise.

There are several other factors which affect post-exercise recovery. These include a balanced and properly executed stretching routine and getting enough quality sleep. While you sleep, your body releases certain hormones which help you to repair and rebuild damaged tissue, and which will directly help your muscles to grow.

Adequate Nutrition is Vital

Post-exercise high-quality nutrition will help your body to repair itself faster, decrease your recovery time, and will help to generally maximise the benefits gained from the exercise. Studies indicate that there is a 30 to 60-minute time-window after exercise when you need to eat, and after which, your body begins to draw upon itself to repair and recover from your exercise session. Drinking enough water is also one of the most important factors in your recovery, as well as for your overall health. This is because your muscles are mostly composed of water.

Since research has shown that post-exercise immunodepression peaks if one exercises for longer than we are technically naturally physically able this becomes an even bigger problem if this scenario is further enhanced due to reduced or inadequate food intake.

The availability of certain key nutrients is vital when recovering from heavy exercise to ensure a robust immune system is maintained and there is enough nutrient to build muscle. Most people mistakenly consume excessive amounts of protein at the expense of other key nutrients such as carbohydrates. Therefore, in doing this they are working against their best interests and overall optimum health.

One of the key nutrients that have been found to help enormously when in recovery from prolonged periods of heavy exercise is carbohydrate. There is a lot of research supporting the hypothesis that carbohydrate is the most important nutritional factor in preventing post-exercise immunodepression. People either conveniently forget or are completely ignorant of the fact that the protein composition of human muscle is typically only somewhere in the region of between 18% and 21% protein and the rest is made up of water, glucose, lipids, and carbohydrates etc.

We will not go into extensive detail here in this section of the book, however, if you want to learn more about this and many other surprising nuggets of useful information about nutrition and exercise then they can be found in The 70 Second Difference book.

Strength, Stamina, Endurance, and Resilience

It is important to understand the difference between strength, stamina and endurance because once understood, you will then be able to devise the most suitable workout routines according to your body type.

Muscular strength is possibly best understood as being a muscle's capacity to exert force against resistance, or weight. This is comparatively easy to measure because your ability to lift a given amount of weight for a single repetition is a good measure of your strength.

Stamina is the length of time at which a muscle, or group of muscles, can perform at or near your maximum capacity. For example, the number of squats you can perform with a given weight which is 90% of your maximum would be a measure of your stamina or the distance which you can carry a similarly heavy object such as an anvil.

Endurance is all about time, and your ability to perform a certain muscular action for a prolonged period regardless of the capacity at which you are working.

Resilience is all about your ability to recover from whatever stresses and demands are placed upon your muscles. However, resilience is mostly all about your state of mind, your mental toughness and ability to endure, perform and deliver under pressure, and about how you recover quickly emotionally.

The muscular composition of your body will always determine how well you will perform at certain sports. The amount of slow twitch muscle fibres you possess will determine how well you perform at endurance-related events, and both type A and type B fast twitch muscle fibres are all about explosive power and your ability to maintain it.

In simple terms, if you possess mostly slow twitch fibres, then you are naturally going to be better suited to endurance sports. Alternatively, if you possess mostly fast twitch muscle fibres, then you are a natural weightlifter. It is important to note, that no matter what your natural predisposition might be in this respect, with the correct training regimen, it is still possible to significantly increase your abilities in your naturally weaker opposing areas of speciality.

Chapter 3: Isometric Exercise Tools

One of the best things about isometric exercise is that if you do not want to use traditional gym equipment or proprietary devices, then you do not have to use them to perform a full workout. Instead, you can either use nothing at all except your own body, immovable objects such as doors, walls, and door jambs, or readily available everyday items. These can include walking sticks/poles, broom handles, towels and sturdy towing, or a climbing rope. I will lay out some of these items as suggestions for alternative equipment/devices you can use for your workout sessions.

Improvised Isometric Exercise Devices
Rope – Either Climbing Rope or Towing Rope

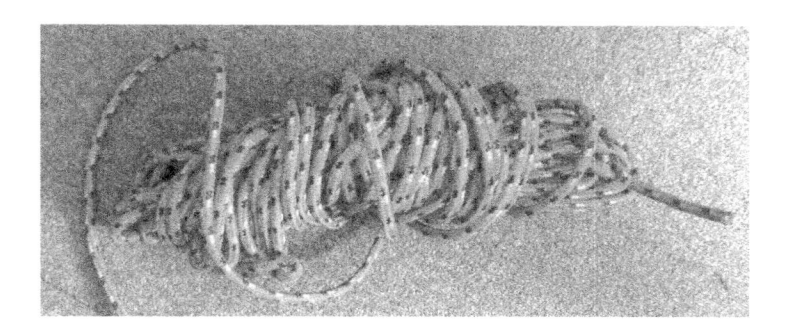

A rope is another simple but highly effective tool that can be used to perform an isometric and/or self-resisted workout routine. the important things to look for in a rope that might be suitable for exercise use are, sufficient length, it must be thick enough to allow a comfortable handgrip, and it must be in good condition so that it will not break during your workout routine.

If you are using your feet to secure the rope, then for added safety and comfort you may wish to loop the rope around the foot as shown. This will make it less likely to slip when it is pulled hard, and it will be more comfortable for the foot as well.

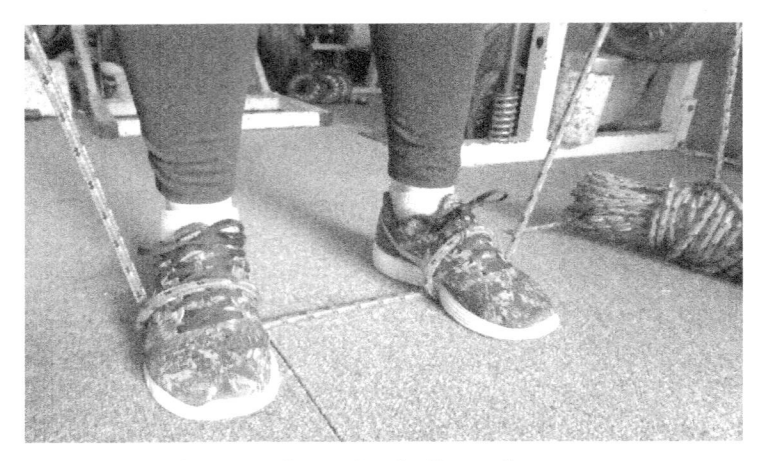

The Humble Beach or Bath Towel

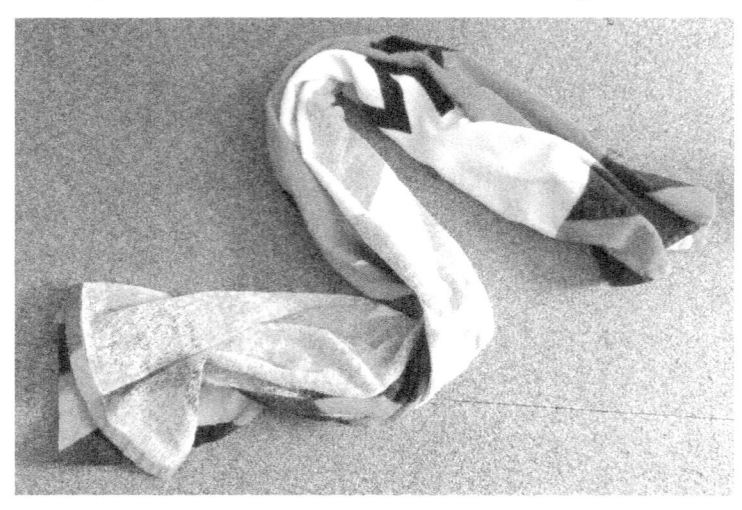

The humble beach or bath towel is a common tool used by isometric enthusiasts who have nothing else to exercise with. It is also an exercise tool of choice for many because it is incredibly versatile. When choosing a towel to exercise with, the important things to look for are that it must be long enough, it must also be flexible enough to enable you to grip it properly, therefore, it must not be too thick. Naturally, it must also be in good condition and not be liable to tear or rip during your exercise session.

The Broom Handle

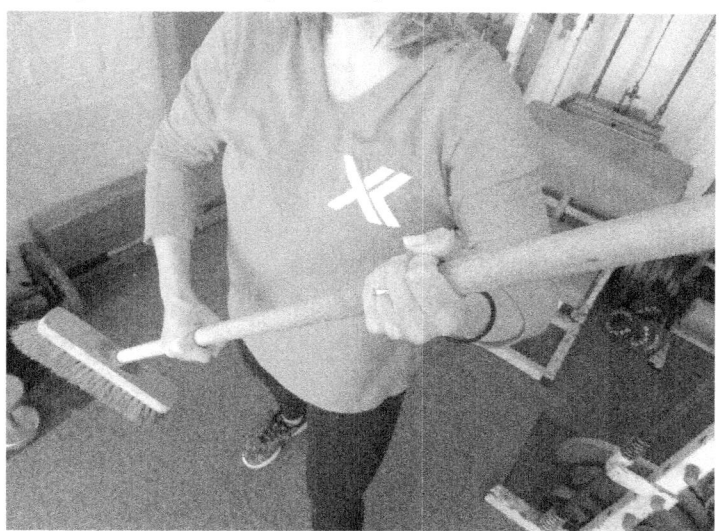

The broom handle can be used almost identically to the walking stick or pro-style walking pole. By its very nature, it is not nearly as flexible as a walking stick or pro-style walking pole. This is because since you can easily take a walking stick or pro-style walking pole virtually anywhere because that is precisely what they have been designed. You would appear to be very odd indeed if you were to carry around a broom with you to exercise with, whereas a walking stick or pro-style walking pole would not look even the slighted bit out of place. If you use a broom handle at home to exercise with, then make sure it is solid and will not break when used in a workout routine. Also, we would strongly caution against using one to support your body weight in any way with the broom handle to support it.

The Walking Stick/Pole

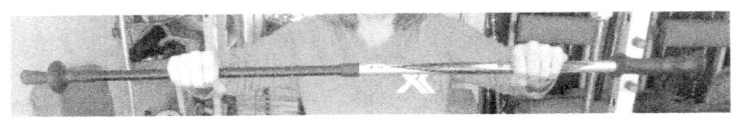

The walking stick or pro-style walking pole is an excellent device to use for an isometric workout. It is an improvised equivalent of a barbell or Bullworker® Classic without the steel cables at each side. One of the great advantages the pro-style walking pole offers is that it can be adjusted to various lengths, which make it easily adaptable for use in a variety of exercises.

Many of the exercises can be performed alone, without any need for partner-assistance. An even greater range of exercises can be performed if a workout partner is available. Nordic Walking Poles are different from ordinary walking poles, but they work equally well for isometric exercises.

Photo: Daniel Case

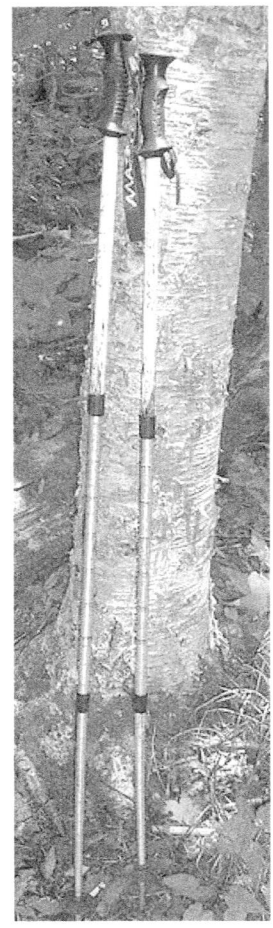

Proprietary Isometric Exercise Equipment

We highly recommend and endorse the Iso-Bow®. as an exercise tool. This inexpensive little device is an amazingly versatile device that allows self-resisted isometric exercises to be performed very easily. It also allows self-resisted isotonic and what I call functional isokinetic exercises to be performed easily. The Iso-Bow® provides the user with a biomechanically sound grip handle which allows almost all exercises to be performed more effectively, and with greater ease and comfort.

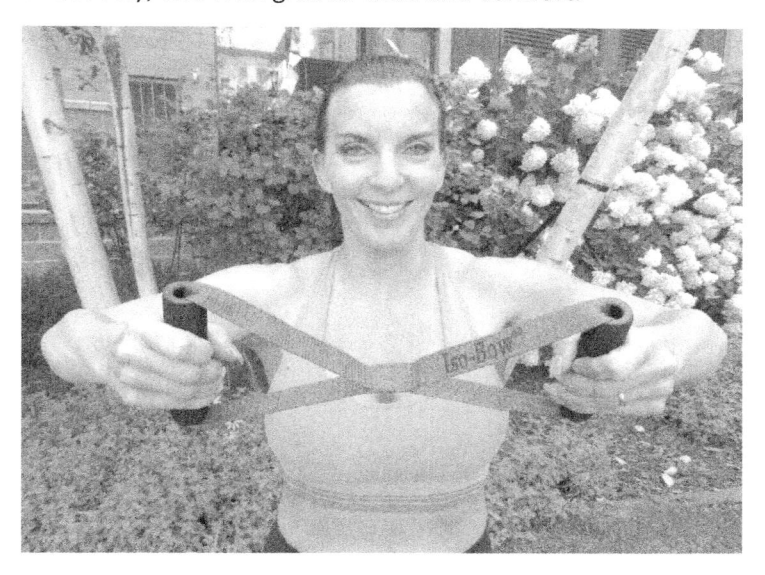

With a pair of Iso-Bows®, you can effectively exercise every major muscle group of the body, and even perform advanced exercises such as the pull-up, the squat, and the deadlift. The level of workout you can get from using a pair of Iso-Bows® can range from an easy low-level beginner's workout, right up to a very high-intensity professional athlete level of workout. Amazingly, you can do all of this without any adjustment being needed to the Iso-Bows®. Each user will benefit proportionately, according to the amount of effort and intensity that is applied during each exercise.

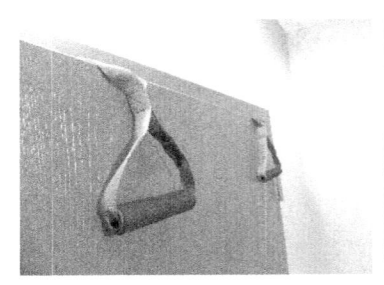

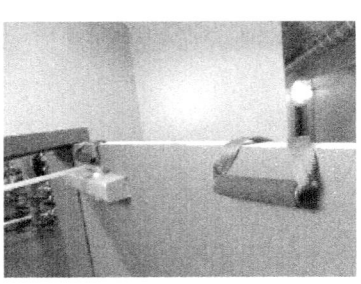

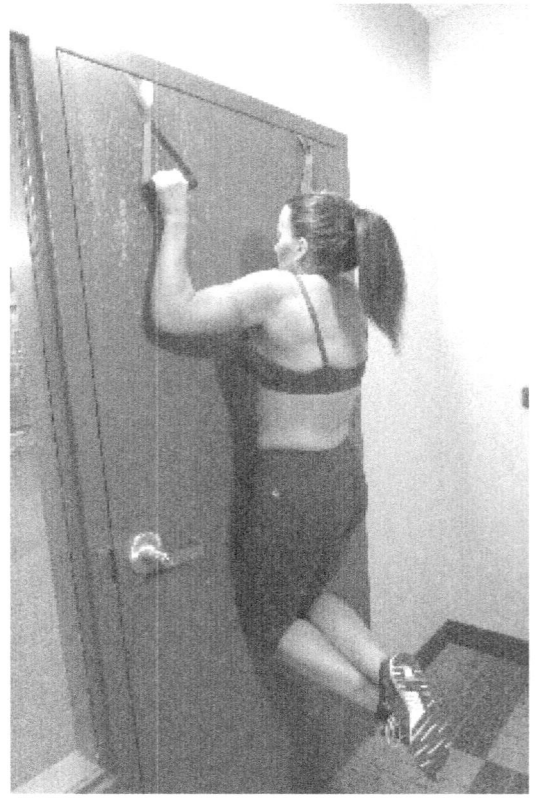

Even a pair of Iso-Bows® are so compact they can easily fit into the average jacket or jeans pocket, a small handbag/purse, a briefcase, or a walking rucksack or bag.

Perhaps the best-known of all isometric/isotonic home exercise devices is the Bullworker® which has been a best-seller when it was launched in the early 1960s. Today, it is still a best-selling device, and with good reason, because it works. The smaller "partner" device is called the Steel Bow®, and both have interchangeable springe so that both men and women of all strength levels and abilities can use them, with roughly equal effectiveness.

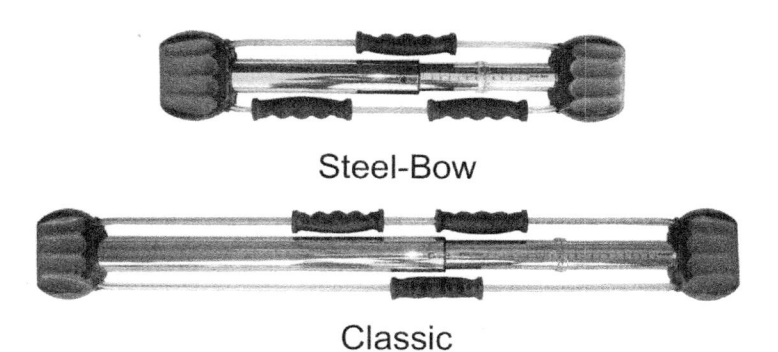

Steel-Bow

Classic

Securing the Iso-Bow® With Your Feet

When performing leg exercises such as squats and lunges, as well as lower back and glute exercises such as the deadlift, it becomes necessary to properly secure the Iso-Bow® using your feet. There are several ways in which the Iso-Bow® can be secured using your feet, and your personal preference of how you do this will depend upon many factors such as your foot size, your choice of footwear, and ease of operation.

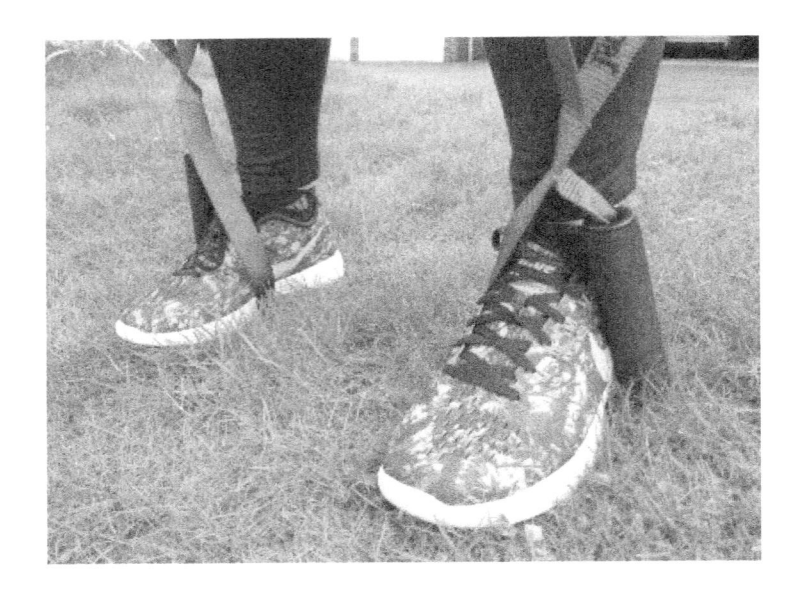

You can secure the Iso-Bow® with your foot inside one of the handles. You do this by adjusting the handgrip to one side, usually the outer side of the foot, and then place your feet inside the loop like a stirrup.

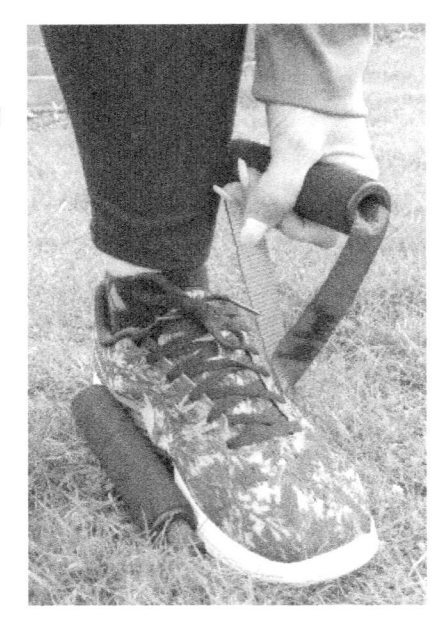

Another method is to place the Iso-Bow® flat on the floor and then stand on one side of the straps so that the handle of the same side sits flush to your inner foot. In this position, it will be your bodyweight combined with the handle pressing against the inner side of your foot which enables you to pull safely and securely.

The final method is to simply place each foot through one end of an Iso-Bow®, stepping onto the foam hand grip as you do so. This method is slightly less stable than the other two methods.

However, if the foot can be pushed far enough through the loop of the Iso-Bow® handle, then the handle will slightly raise the level of your heel making it easier for some people to squat or lunge.

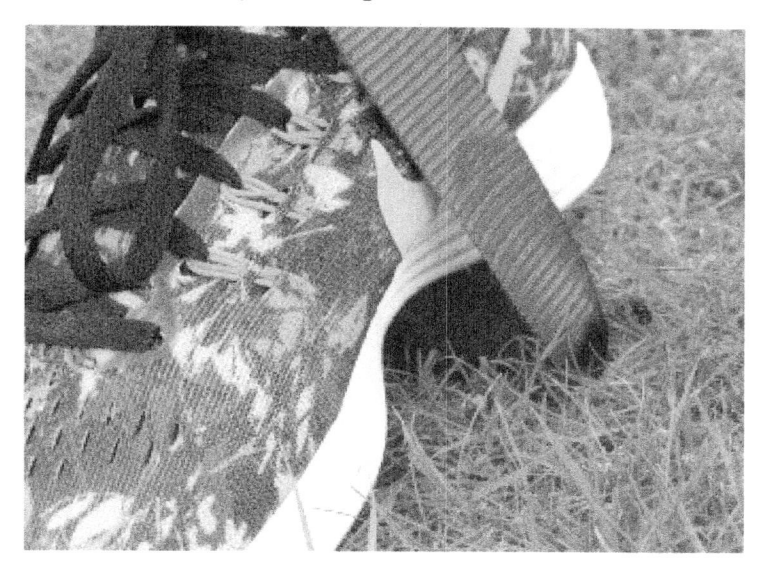

Naturally, safety is always a top priority so whichever method you ultimately choose to use, you should always make sure that when securing the Iso-Bow® with your feet that there is never any chance of it slipping in any way while you exercise.

Chapter 4: How Effective is a 10x7 Second Total-Body Workout? And About the Exercise Model

Helen Renée is an American who is married to a Brit. She was born in Minnesota and grew up in Northern Alaska after her father became an Ice Road Trucker.

Helen went from being 40 lbs overweight to contest-winning condition almost effortlessly in less than 6 months and with workout sessions lasting no longer than 10 minutes per day.

Helen is an isometric exercise expert instructor and champion Bikini Fitness Athlete who achieved spectacular contest-winning results after meeting her exercise scientist husband.

Helen's husband is one of the world's leading experts on isometric exercise, plant-based nutrition, and was a former coach to the 4-times World's Strongest Man, Jon Pall Sigmarsson of Iceland.

Currently, Helen has co-authored 21 fitness books and since she and her husband share a common fascination with mysteries and the paranormal, they have co-authored a best-selling book on the subject.

Since meeting and marrying her British husband they have enjoyed a joyous journey together discovering the many differences between the two countries which share a common language and culture.

They began writing these stories and anecdotes down and very soon had enough to produce a fun-filled and light-hearted book about what it is like Being American Married to a Brit.

Helen is remarkably strong with the exceptional power-to-weight ratio one would expect from a former gymnast.

She is also an isometric and TRISOmetric™ exercise instructor, consultant, and instructor-trainer for TWiEA™ The World Isometric Exercise Association.
www.TWiEA.com – www.HelenRenee.com

The following pictures are of Helen Renée taken in January 2015 before she started performing a daily 10 x 7-second total-body exercise isometric exercise routine.

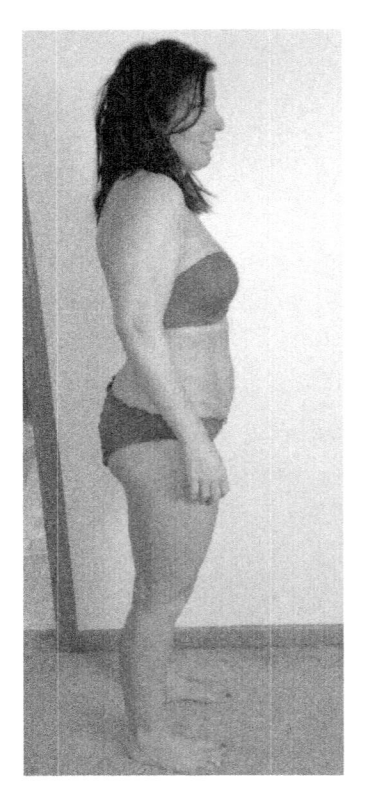

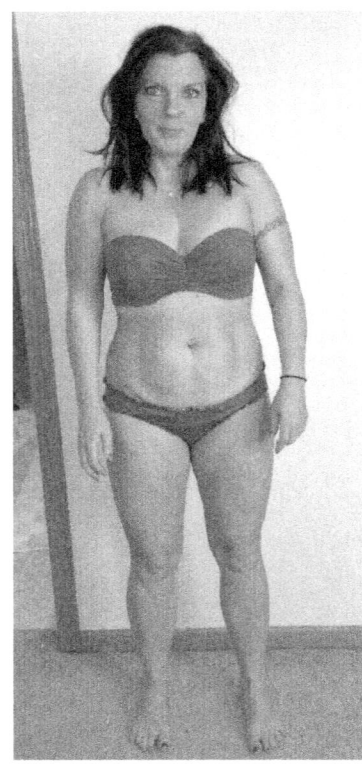

The following pictures are of Helen Renée 1-year later, in January 2016. She became a contest-winning Bikini Fitness competitor within 1-year of daily isometric exercise training lasting only minutes each day. Now, Helen only trains using only isometric exercises because they are so effective. She simply exercises regularly each day and applies more intensity to each exercise than a normal person would who simply wanted to get a little stronger, fitter and maintain a good overall body shape. Helen also eats sensibly.

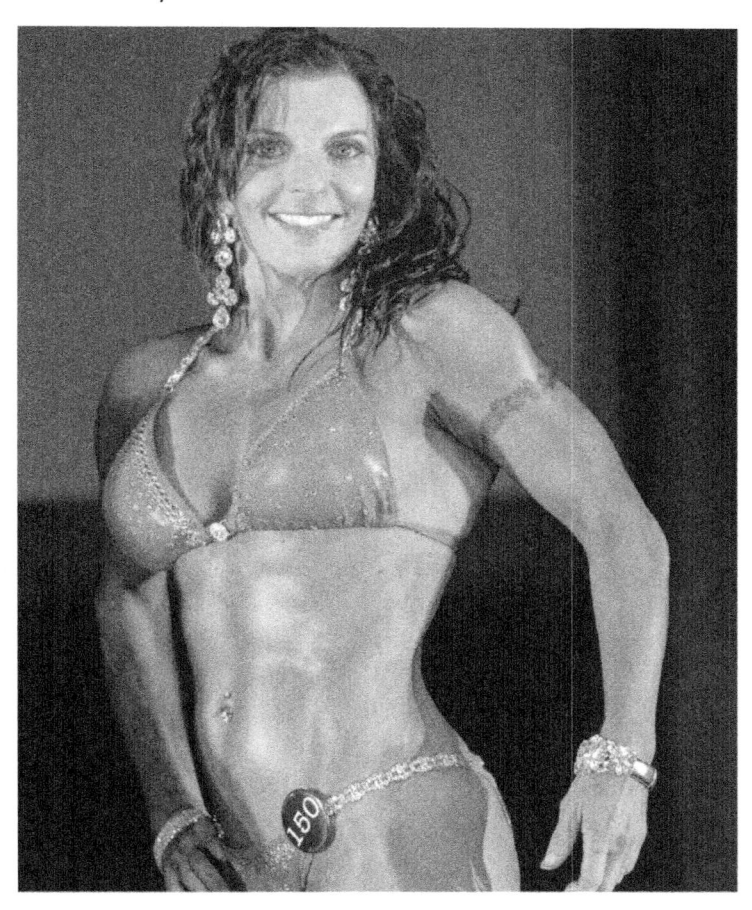

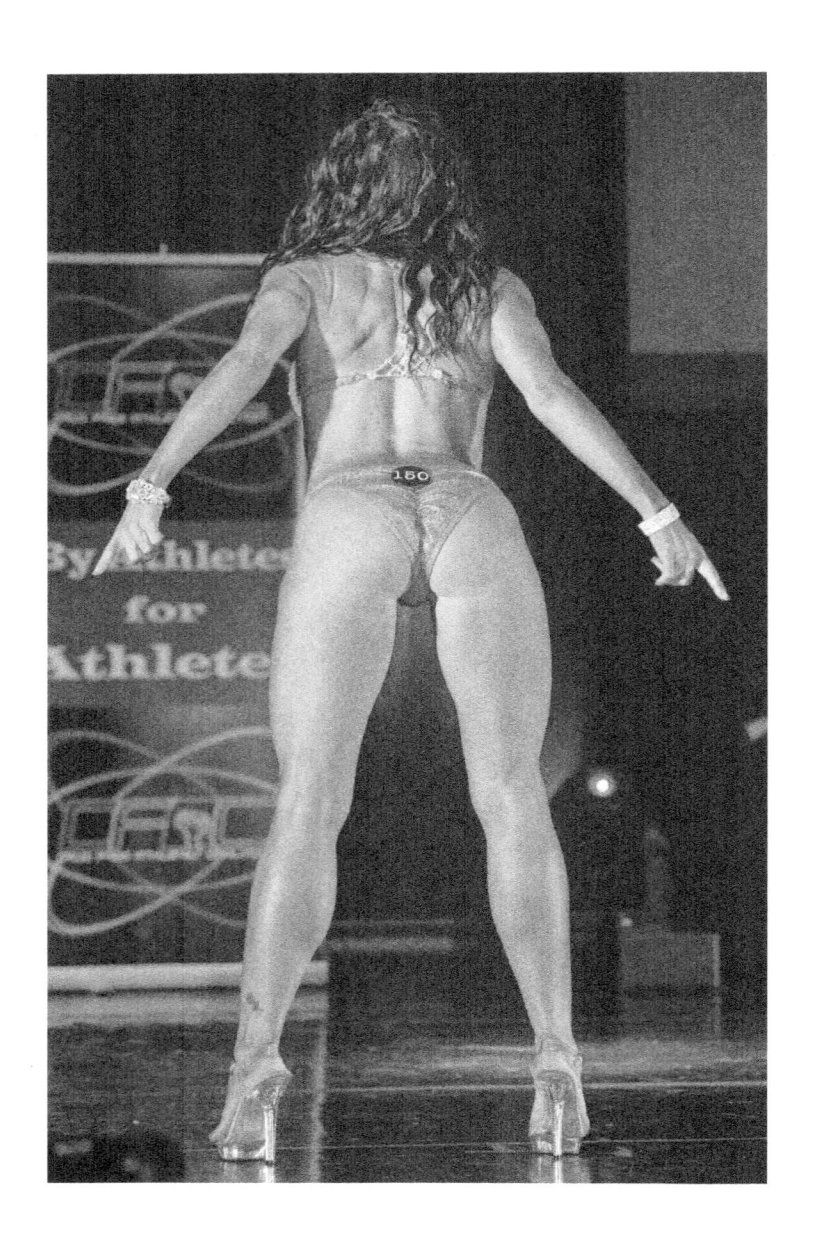

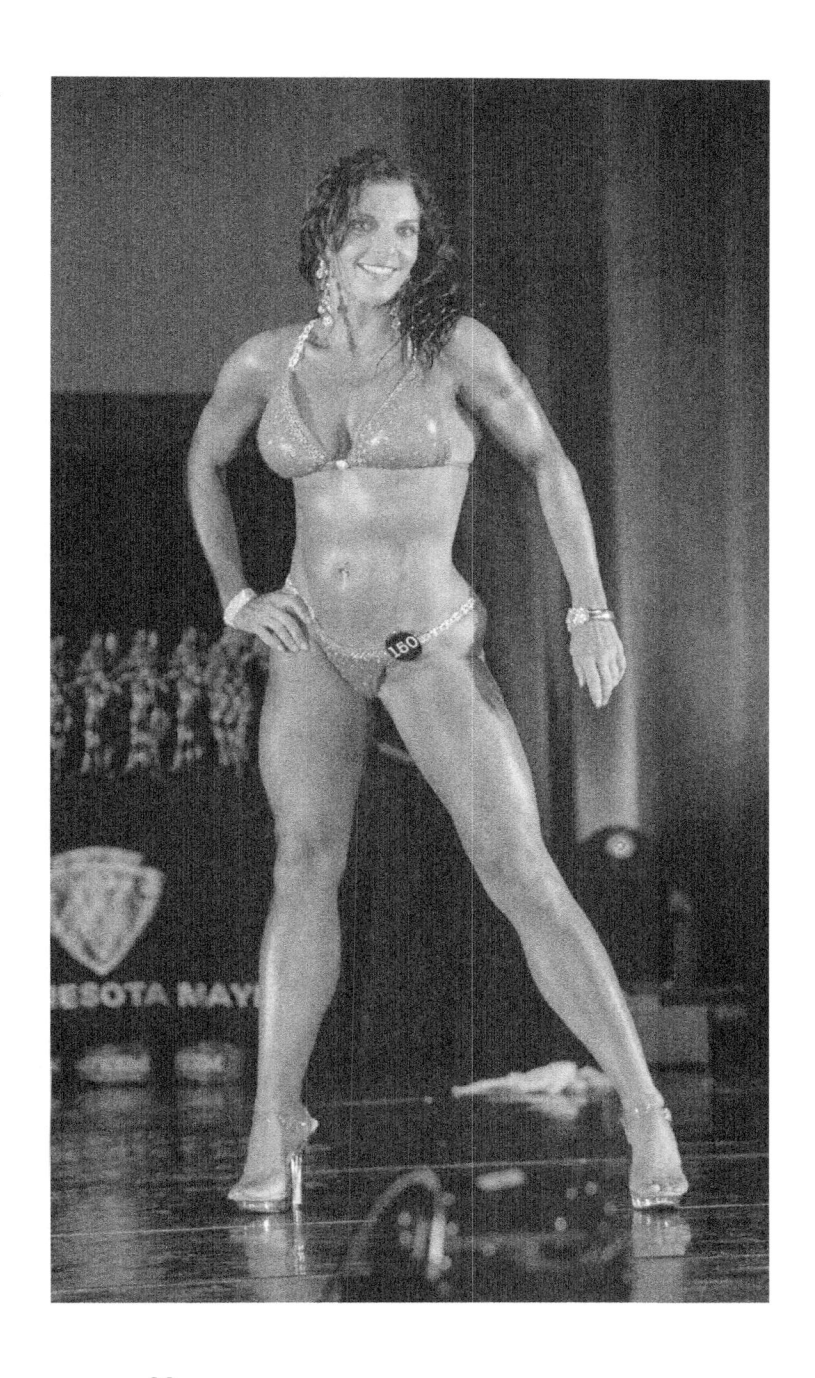

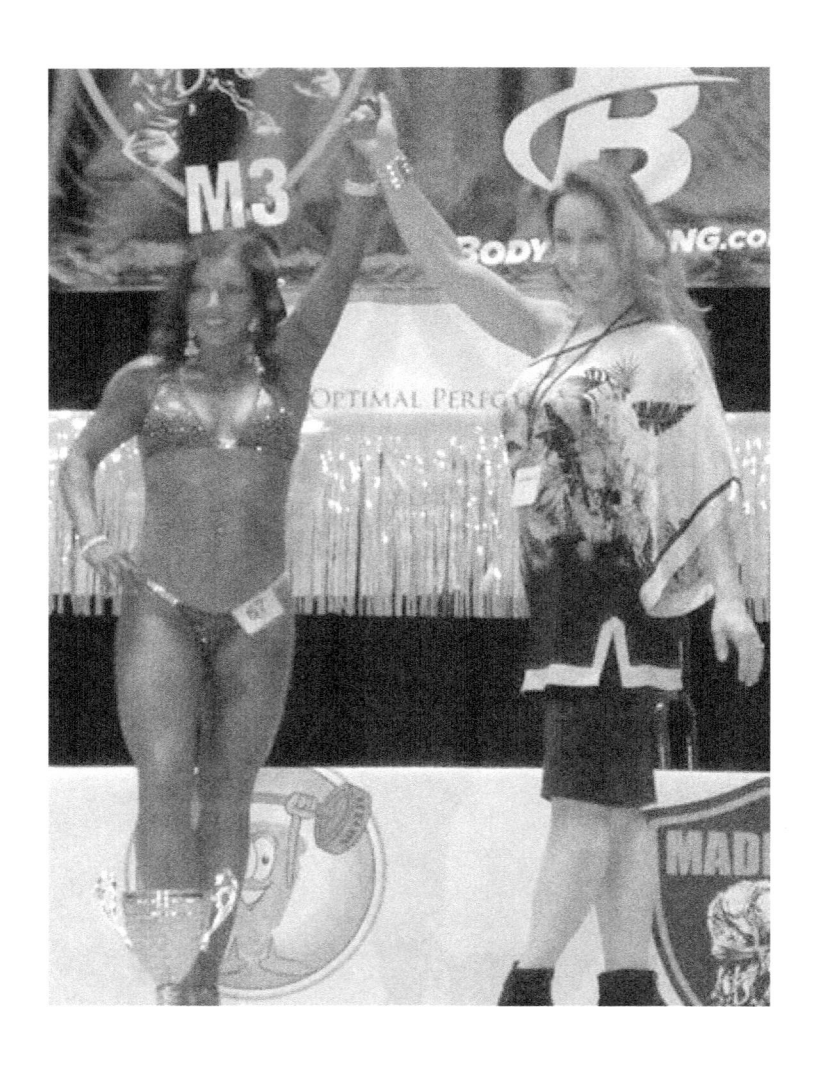

The Author and an Isometric Experiment

The following picture is of my arm taken in December 2016. This was the result of a year-long experiment to see what results could be gained through a basic high-intensity isometric exercise routine using only the minimum number of exercises.

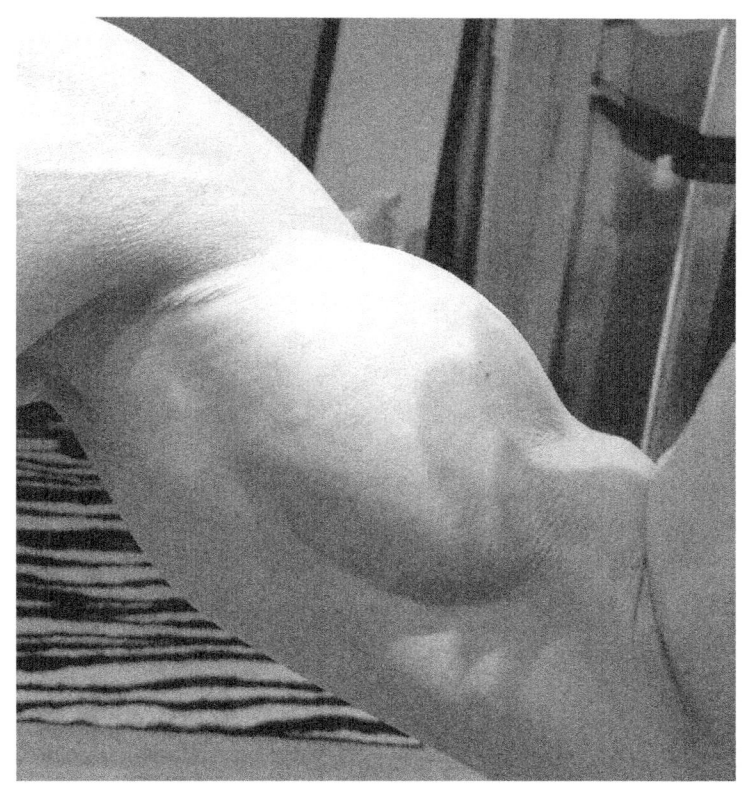

My arm after 1 year of basic isometric maintenance training. This picture was taken to record the results of the experiment in December 2016.
The routine allowed just 1 x 7-second isometric exercise per muscle/muscle group per day at a target level of applied force/intensity of between 75% and 80%.

For one year, starting in January 2016, I performed a daily 10 exercise x 7-second total-body isometric routine. It is common for even the most experienced athletes to count the elapsed exercise time increasingly quickly, almost in direct proportion to an increasing level of applied force/intensity.

Therefore, I typically aimed to perform a 10-second isometric hold for each exercise, and this way I would always reach the desired goal of 7-seconds in good style.

My target level of intensity for each exercise was around 75-80%, slightly higher than the typically recommended average of two thirds, or 66.6%. However, this still effectively meant that I exercised each of my biceps for a total of between just 21 and 30 seconds per week, nothing more.

Amazingly, at the end of the year-long experiment I achieved an improvement in both the strength and size of each arm, albeit slight. Even though I am well-versed in the science of isometrics I still found it remarkable because it was in exchange for a maximum of 30 seconds per week of exercise time. Once again, this only served to reinforce the fact that the best results are always gained through pin-point focus, high intensity, and by never confusing activity with accomplishment.

Chapter 5:
Things to Remember Before You Begin

- The first and perhaps the most important thing to remember is: **NEVER HOLD YOUR BREATH AT ANY TIME.**
- Breathing in and out naturally during all isometric exercises will also help you count the number of elapsed seconds much more accurately, with one full breath in and out taking approximately one second.
- We recommend that you read the instructions about each exercise carefully. You can also watch the associated videos via the TWiEA™ website if you wish to become a member and access the resource.
- Always leave a safe distance between you and others if exercising with any proprietary device or IIED (Improvised Isometric Exercise Device)
- Always check the structural integrity of any type of exercise device. If there is any doubt about the structural integrity, then do not use it for exercise or any other purpose.
- Double-check that any/all adjustable joints on the exercise device and/or IIED are secure before use.
- Weight loss/fat loss will ONLY occur when any exercise plan is used in conjunction with a calorie-controlled diet.
- It is critically important to completely focus your mind on the exercise being performed. Envision the muscle you are exercising is growing larger and stronger.

- ⚠ Always consult a professional coach to devise a detailed stretching routine, this will ensure that you are stretching the areas effectively rather than risking injury.
- ⚠ Always ensure that a stable line of biomechanical progression is achieved before engaging in and performing any exercise.
- ⚠ Warming-up, stretching, and cooling down are three of the most overlooked yet essential elements to exercise, and we cannot stress their importance strongly enough.
- ⚠ During ANY form of physical exercise, including isometrics, if you apply too much intensity too soon, then you may inadvertently strain a muscle. Isometric exercise is particularly intense, and a single isometric exercise engages a great many more muscle fibres than even high-intensity weight training, and isometrics engages the muscle fibres at a much higher level too.

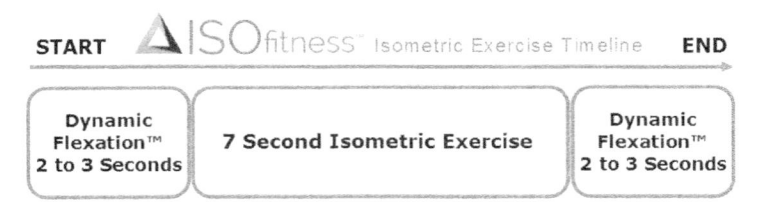

START ⚠ISOfitness™ Isometric Exercise Timeline **END**

| Dynamic Flexation™ 2 to 3 Seconds | 7 Second Isometric Exercise | Dynamic Flexation™ 2 to 3 Seconds |

For safety's sake, we always recommend using Dynamic Flexation™ to engage your muscles gradually and progressively into ANY exercise, especially isometrics, according to what we call The ISOfitness Exercise Engagement Timeline™.

The main benefit to properly warming up for several minutes before a workout is injury prevention, and to increase your heart rate and the circulation to your muscles, ligaments, and tendons. It is important to remember that warming-up and stretching are two different concepts and that stretching is not a good warm-up. This is because stretching will put the muscle in an un-contracted position and weaken it. Stretching is always best performed after a workout has been completed, together with a proper cool-down. In addition to properly warming-up, always perform a gentle flex and stretch of the muscles and joints which are about to be exercised. For example, squatting down fully to flex the thighs and loosen the knees is always a good idea before performing any leg exercises. Dynamic Flexation™ performed before any exercise should help to ensure greater great flexibility and increased blood supply to the muscles and surrounding tissue.

Isometric exercises are deceptively powerful. Even when engaging in what may feel like only moderate-intensity exercise, you are probably still engaging and contracting many more muscle fibres than you would in a similar isotonic exercise. Therefore, if you are in any doubt whatsoever, then always perform the exercise with a little less intensity.

All exercises and workout plans work equally well for men and women. Both sexes can build strength, muscle, body build, or simply get into great shape if so desired, each according to their natural ability.

In our exercise resource books, the exercises listed are suggestions of what can be performed for each body part/muscle group. We are not suggesting that they should all be performed. Instead, users may wish to select the most suitable exercises from each section. In our course books, please perform the exercises according to the workout session notes.

Only perform 10 exercises, which is one for each muscle group/body part. If there are other exercises demonstrated for the same muscle group/body part, then these are only shown as possible variations for future use to keep the routine interesting and varied. A variation exercise is a substitute exercise, not an additional one.

Finally, please read, review, and ensure that you have fully complied with all recommendations in the section entitled: 'Important General Safety and Health Guidelines,' and only start using the isometric, or any exercise system with the full approval of your physician.

The Essential Feel Better in 70 Seconds 10x7 Second Exercise Workout Routine Overview

1) Abdominal Knee Raise and Trunk Curl

2 & 3) Biceps and Triceps Dual Self-Resistance (Left and Right Side)

4) Back: Upper Chest-Level Pull-Apart

5) Lower Back: Lying Shoulder and Legs Raise

6) Chest: Palm-Press Together

7) Shoulders: Side Lateral Raise Hands Interlock

8) Upper Thighs Front: Wall Squat

9) Upper Thigh Hamstring: Wall Hamstring Curl

10) Calf: Immovable Object Heel Raise-Push

Chapter 6:

The Feel Better in 70 Seconds 10x7 Second Exercise Workout Routine

1) Abdominal Knee Raise and Trunk Curl

Sit on a chair or any other solid object or lean back against a solid wall, place the palms of both hands face downwards over the top of one knee. Then, curl your body forwards and downwards by contracting the abdominals, and at the same time, raise the knee resisted by your hands.

When you perform an isometric exercise never hold your breath. Always breathe deeply and naturally, which will be about 10 full breaths in and out at a rate of about 1 second per full breath. Perform each exercise for no less than 7 seconds, and no longer than 10.

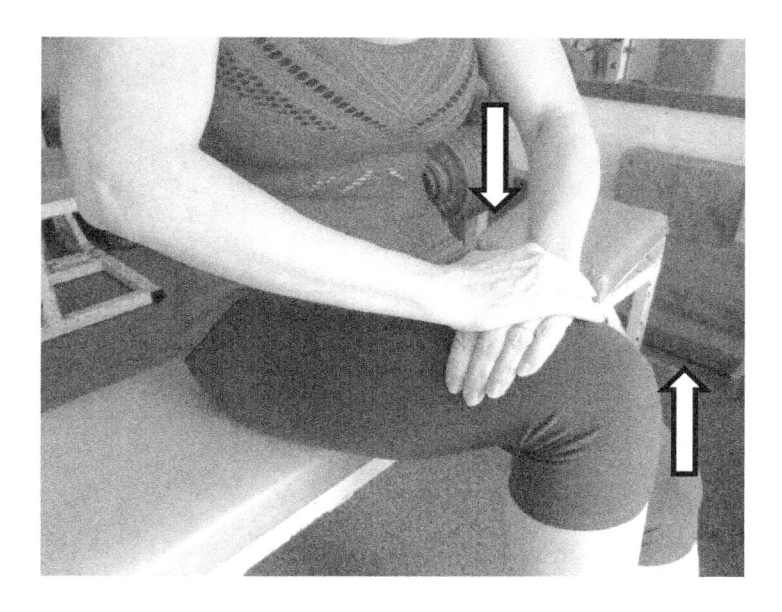

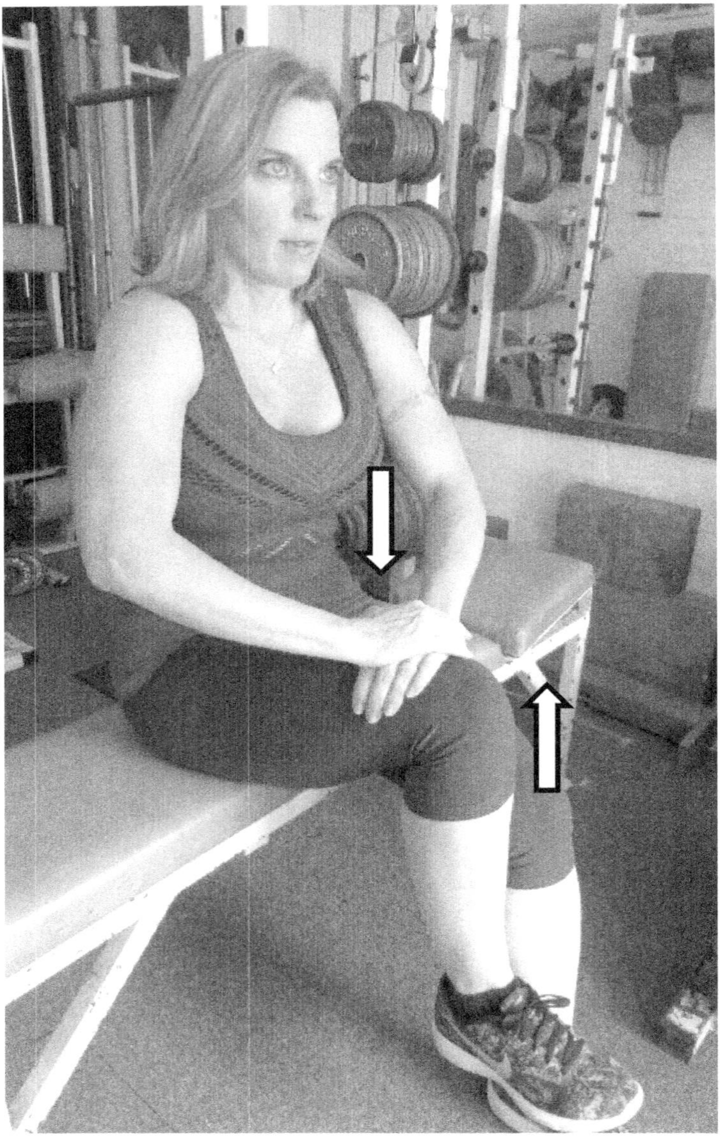

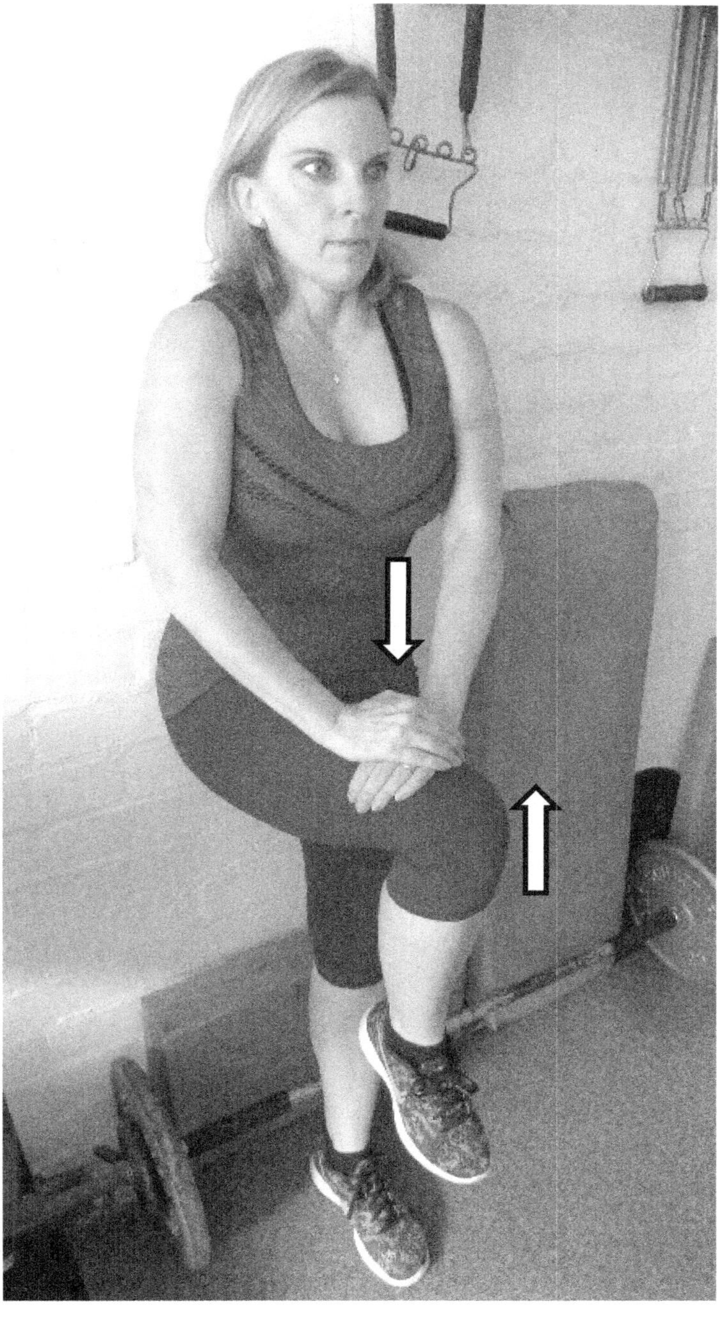

2 & 3) Biceps and Triceps Dual Self-Resistance (Left and Right Side)

The biceps and triceps dual resistance technique will exercise the biceps muscles on one arm, while at the same time exercising the triceps muscles on the other arm. One arm, with the palms of the hands facing downwards, interlocks hands with the other arm with palms facing upwards.

Both arms and elbows must always remain close to the body, with elbows bent to allow the muscles to be exercised properly. A lower interlocking hand position will exercise the muscles in the lower range, a mid-point hand position will exercise the middle range, and a high-point hand position will exercise the upper range.

When you perform an isometric exercise never hold your breath. Always breathe deeply and naturally, which will be about 10 full breaths at a rate of about 1 second per breath. Perform each exercise for no less than 7 seconds, and no longer than 10.

Note: Some people prefer to perform this exercise with the hands positioned roughly along the midline at the front of the body, or with alternate hands/arms at opposing sides of the body. Both methods are fine, and it is more important to find a position that works best for you.

Never allow your wrists to bend backwards during any exercise as this reduces the level of intensity that can be applied. Also, remember to change from palms up to palms down on each hand/side to exercise the biceps and triceps of both arms.

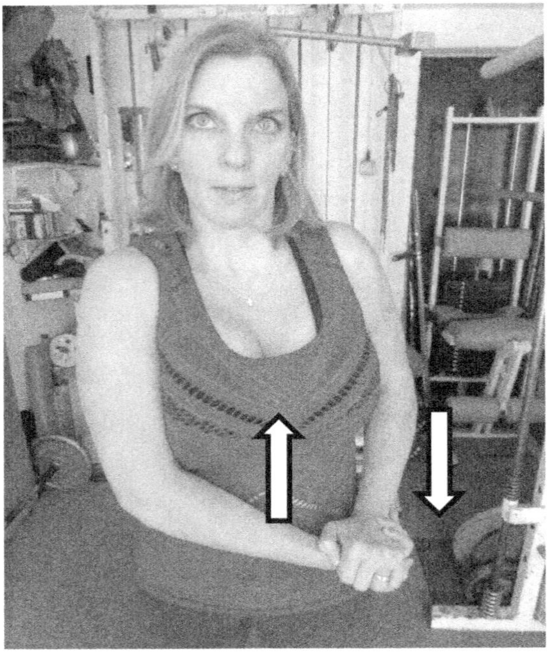

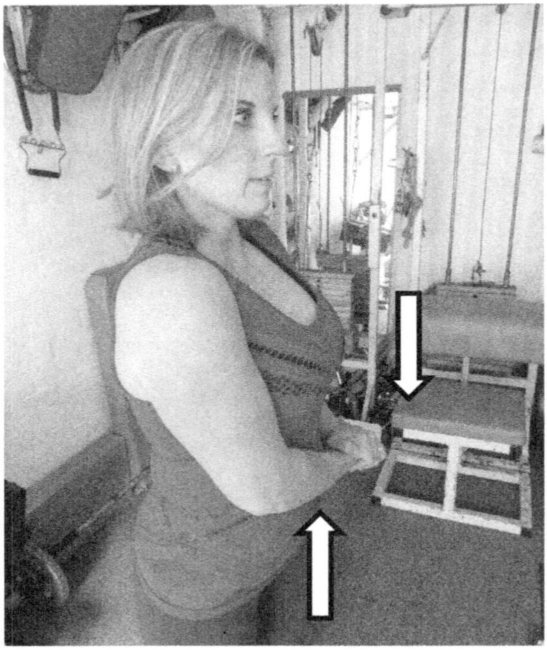

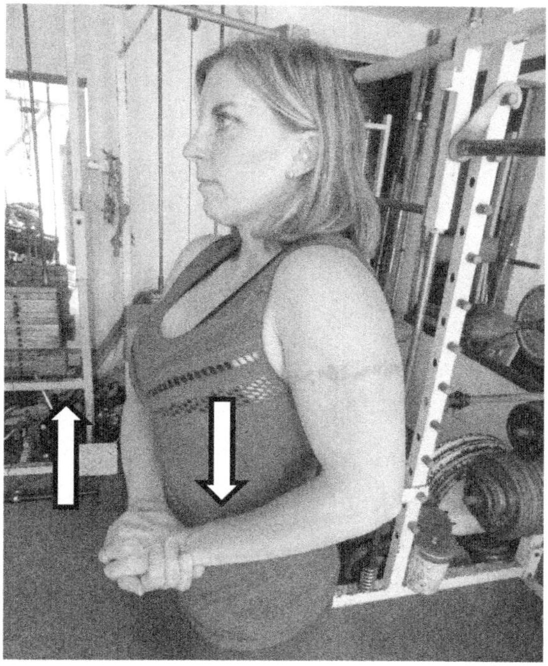

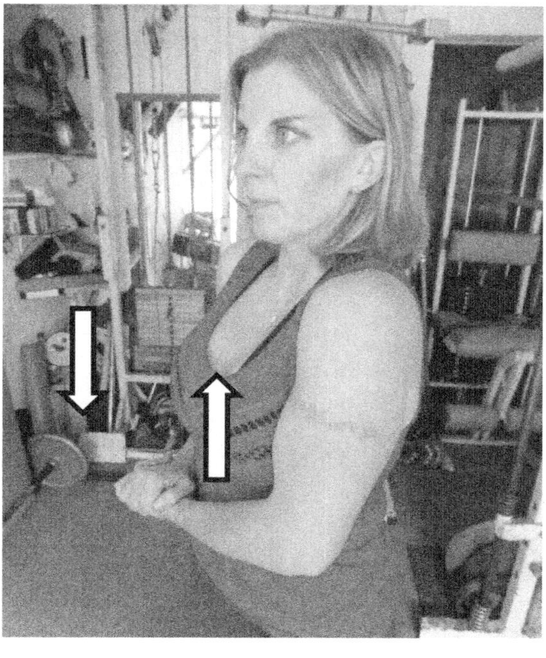

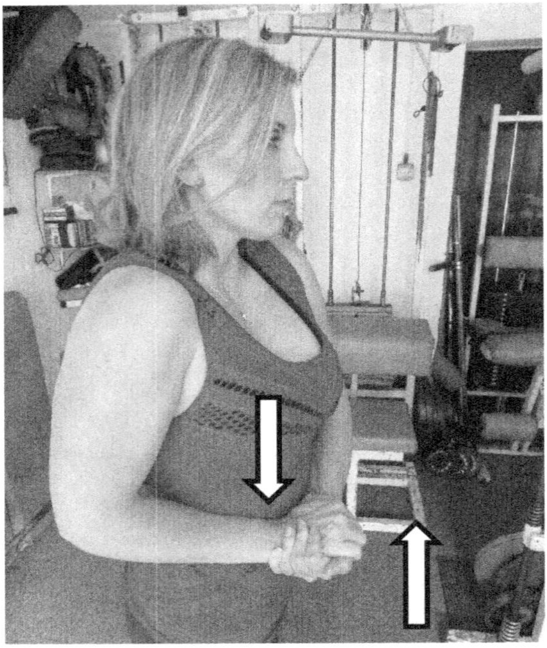

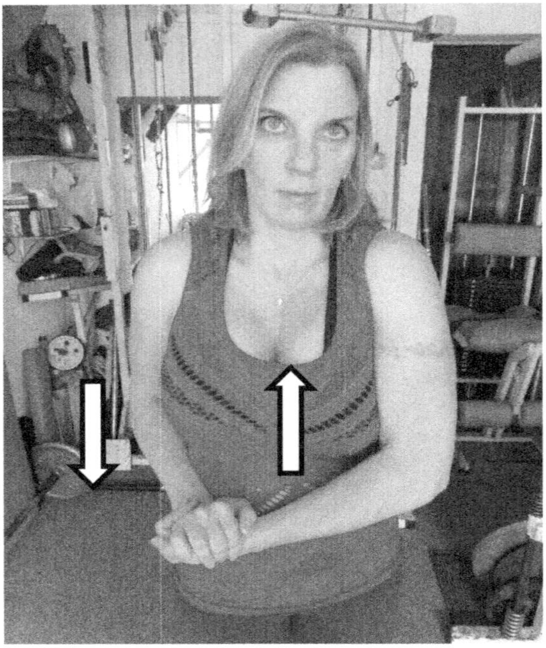

Variation Arms: Biceps and Triceps Dual Resistance with Rope

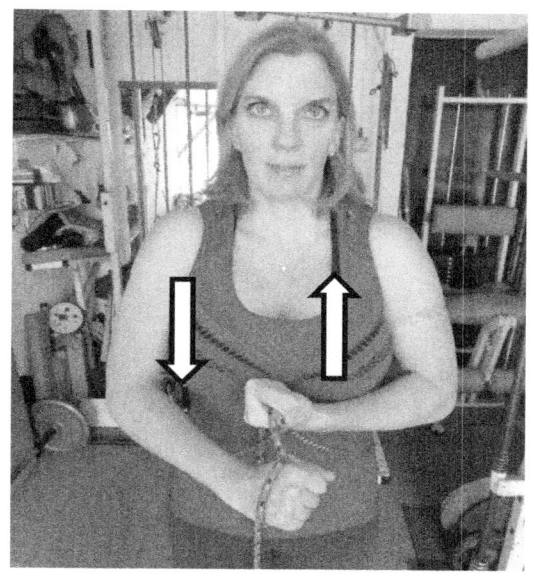

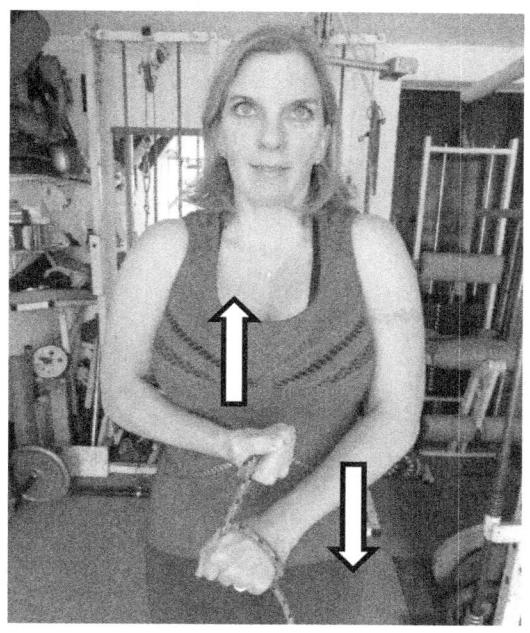

Variation Arms: Biceps and Triceps Dual Resistance with a Towel

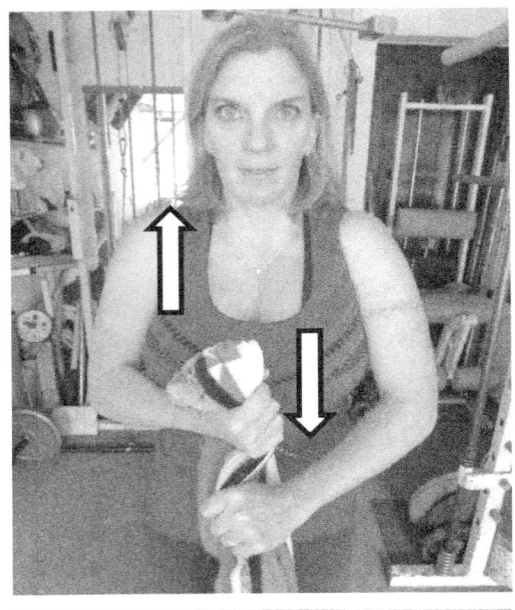

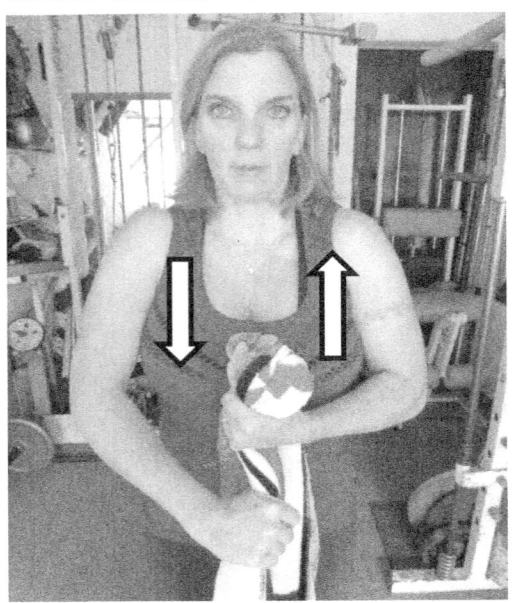

Variation Arms: Biceps and Triceps Dual Resistance with Iso-Bow® - Long Bow

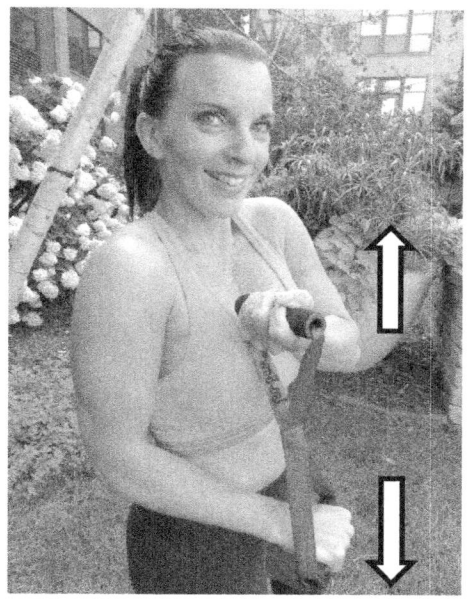

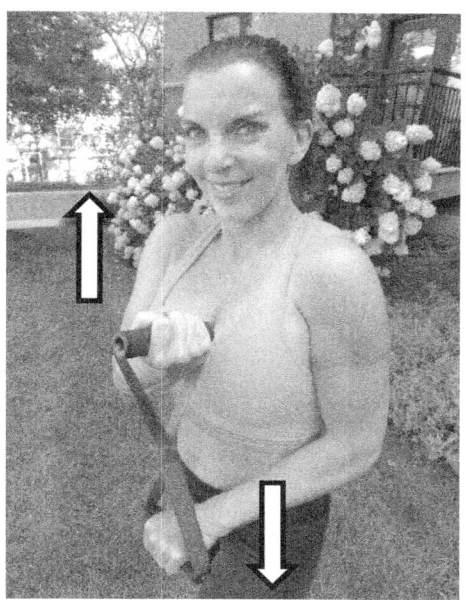

Variation Arms: Biceps and Triceps Dual Resistance with Iso-Bow® - Short Bow

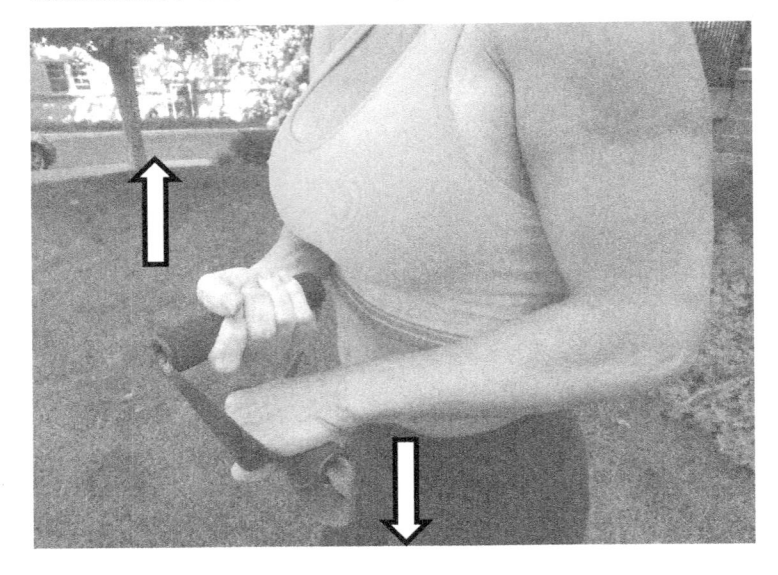

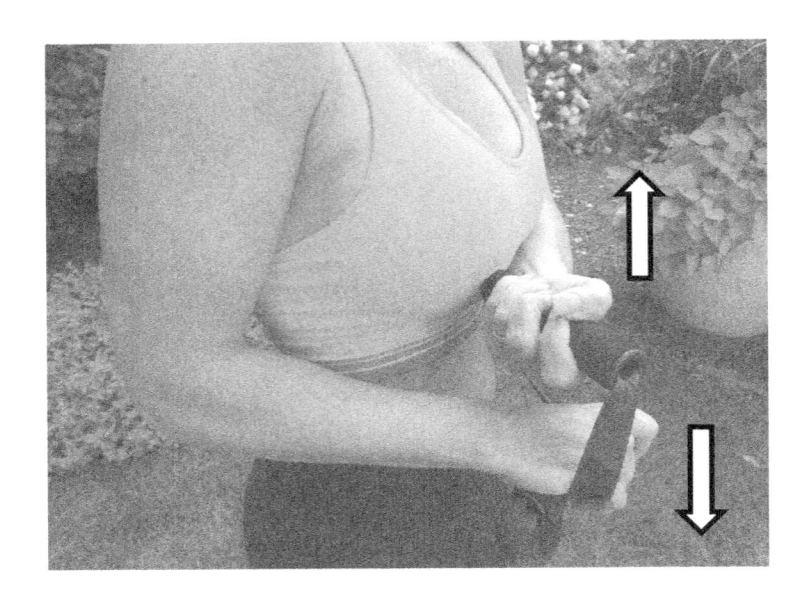

4) Back: Upper Chest-Level Pull-Apart

In either a seated or a standing position with your torso upright raise your bent arms out sideways until they are roughly parallel to the floor. Inter-hook your fingers together or use any other solid grip that will not slip.

If you are using rope or a towel, then make sure you grip it securely. You can loop the rope around your hands if needed. An Iso-Bow® or similar will provide you with the best grip.

In this position, apply tension as if to pull your hands apart, which your grip prevents from happening, as you engage the upper back, shoulder, and neck muscles.

When you perform an isometric exercise never hold your breath. Always breathe deeply and naturally, which will be about 10 full breaths at a rate of about 1 second per breath.

Perform each exercise for no less than 7 seconds, and no longer than 10.

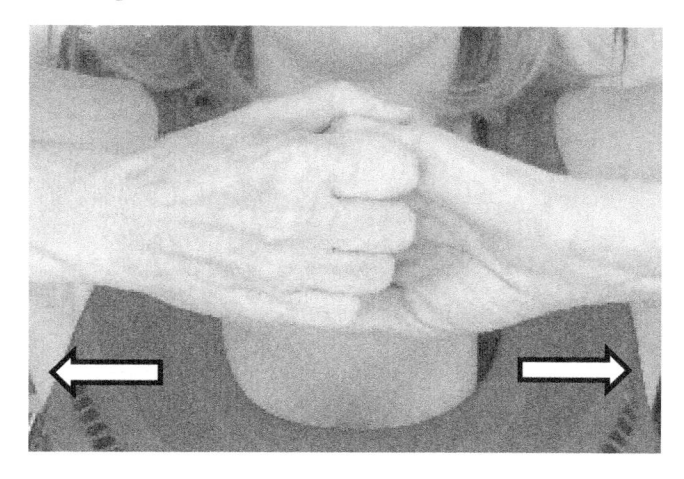

101

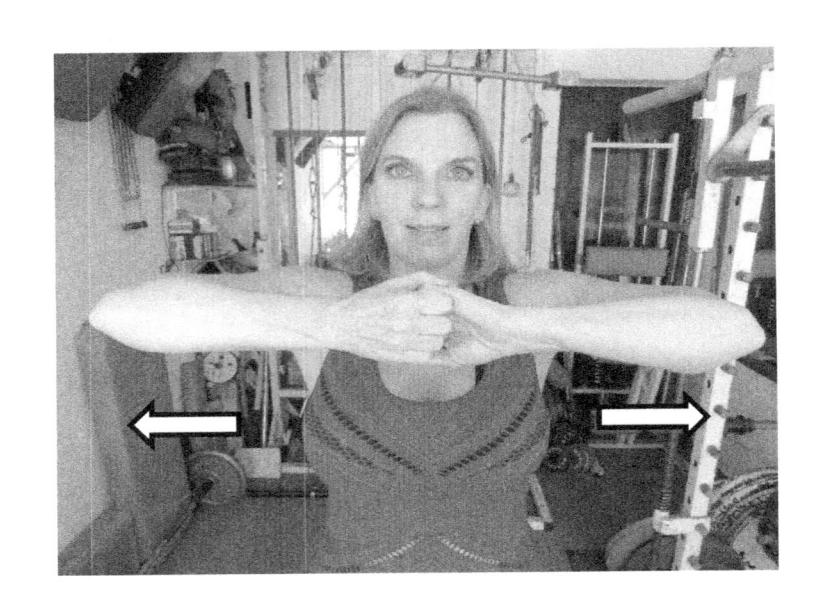

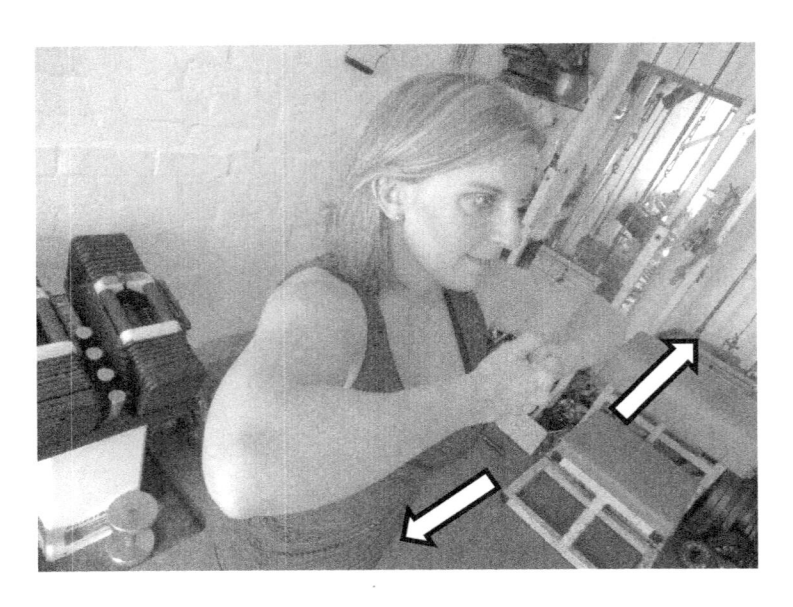

Variation Upper Back: Pull-Apart with Rope

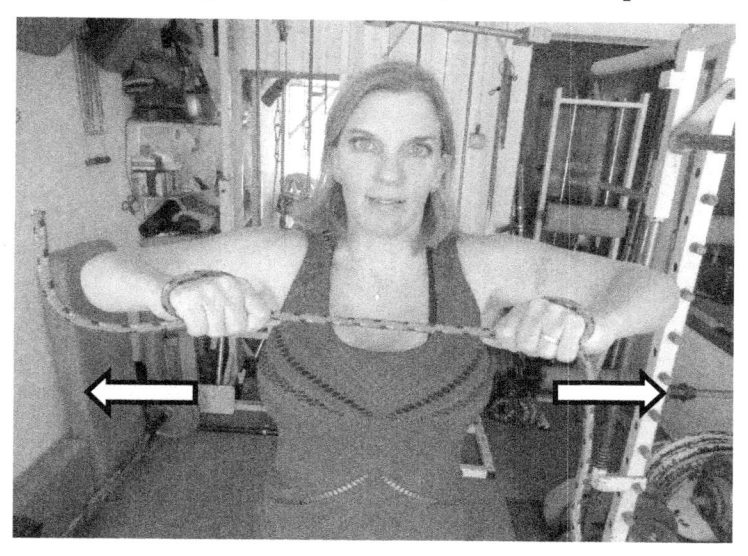

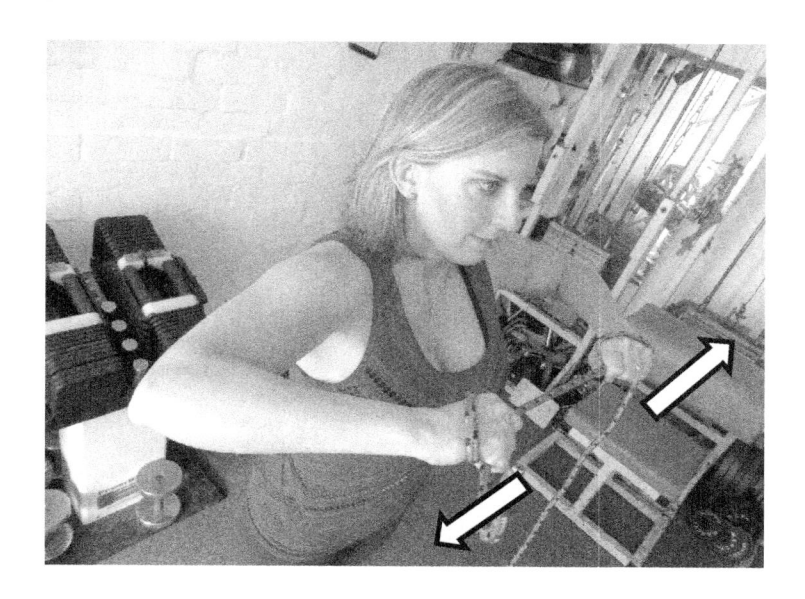

102

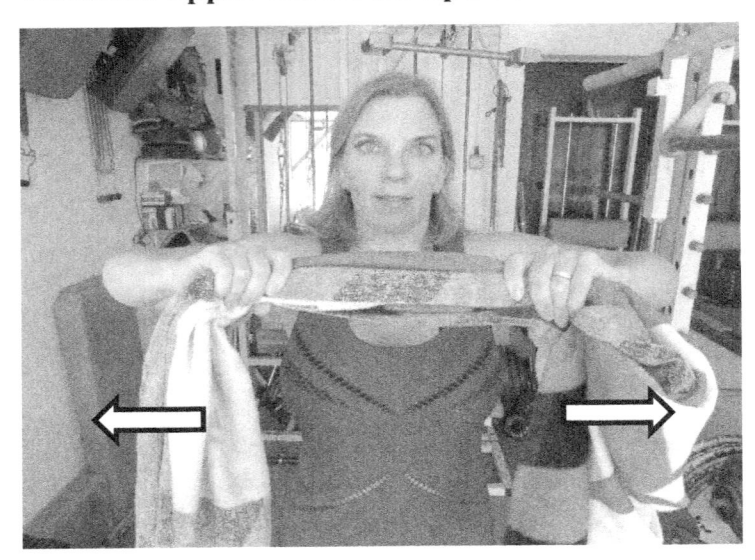

Variation Upper Back: Pull-Apart with Towel

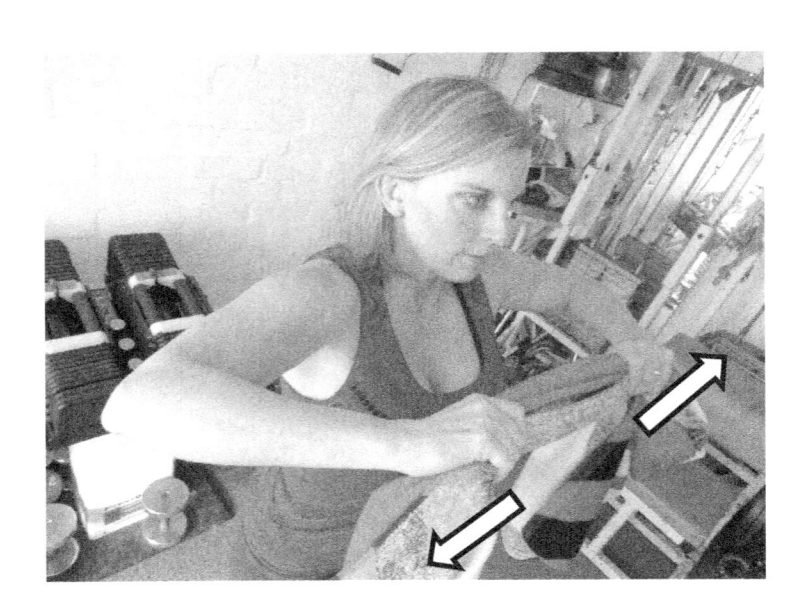

Variation Upper Back: Pull-Apart Iso-Bow®

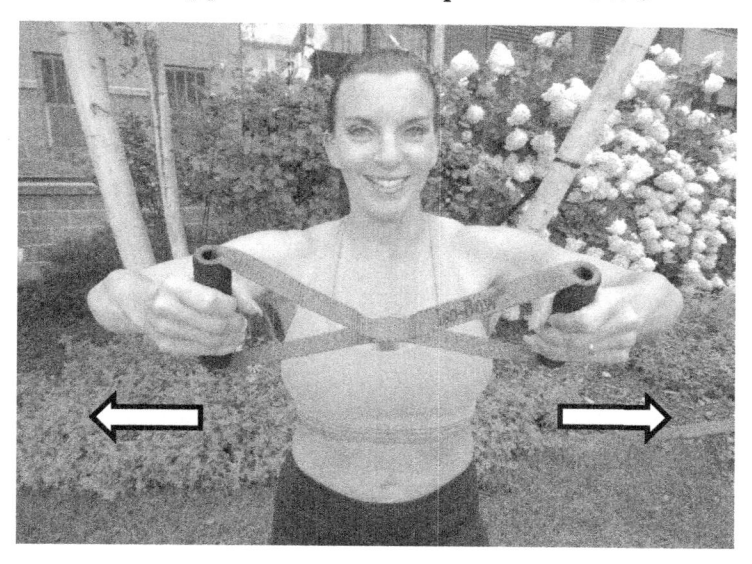

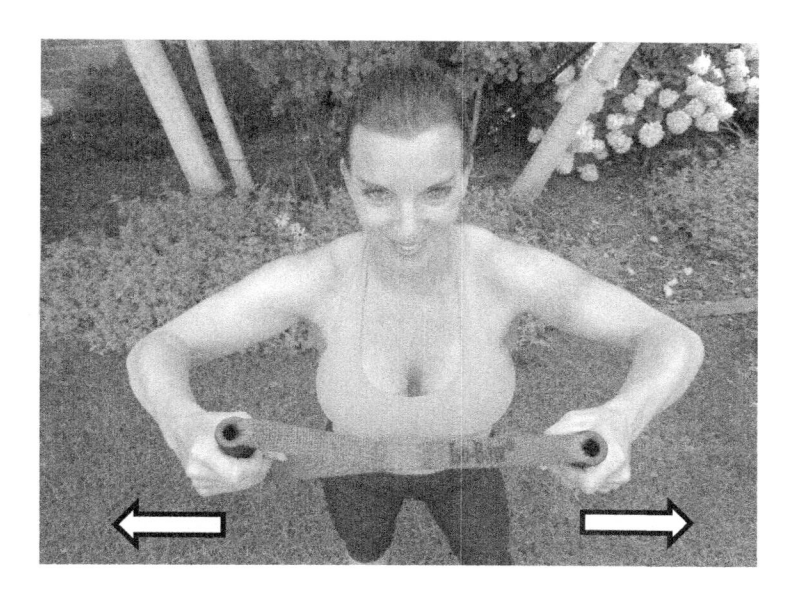

5) Lower Back: Lying Shoulder and Legs Raise

Lay full-length face down on the floor, preferably on an exercise mat. Keep your arms to your side and legs and feet together.

Slowly raise your shoulders feet and thighs/legs off the floor simultaneously to the highest position you can comfortably reach to perform the exercise.

When you perform an isometric exercise never hold your breath.

Always breathe deeply and naturally, which will be about 10 full breaths at a rate of about 1 second per breath.

Perform each exercise for no less than 7 seconds, and no longer than 10.

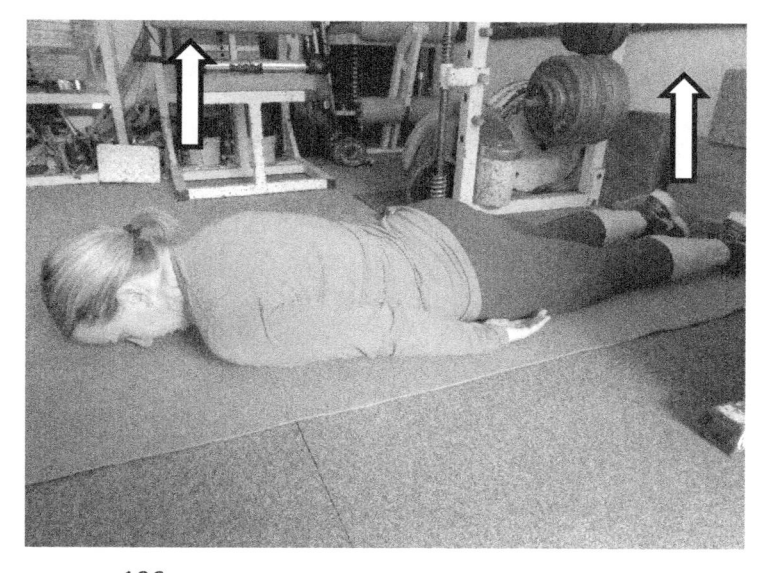

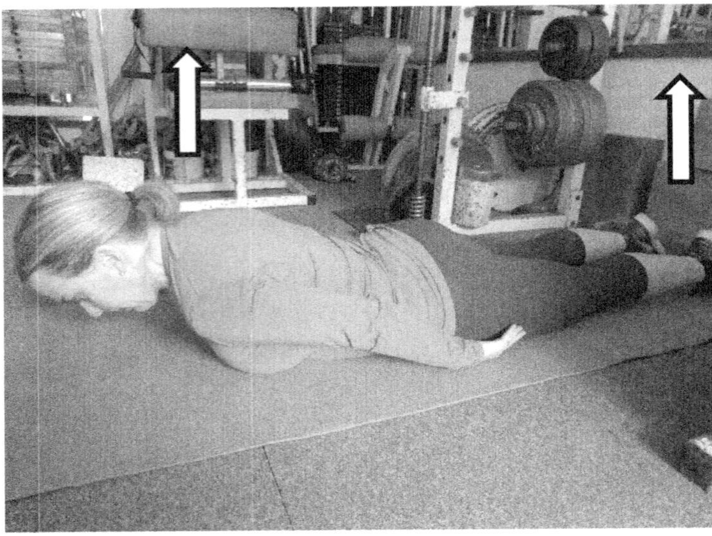

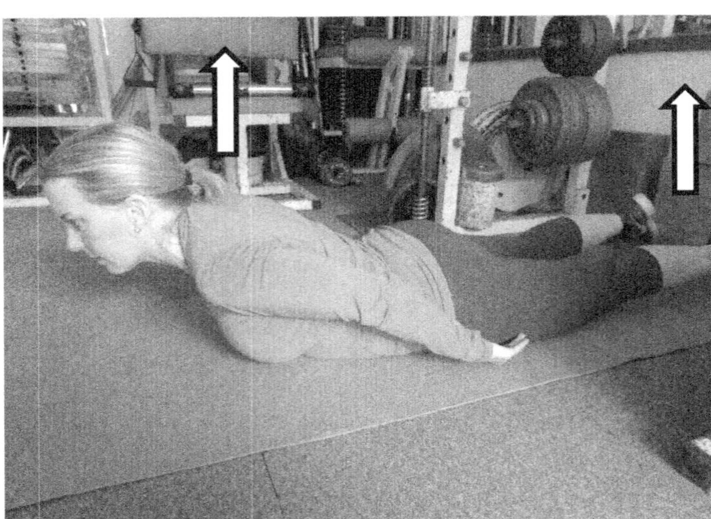

Variation Lower Back: Deadlift with Rope

Stand with your feet roughly shoulder-width apart in an appropriate place along a length of sturdy rope.

Make sure that the rope is right in the middle of your foot, under your arches to help ensure the rope will not slip out. Bend and squat slightly down from your knees and hips, keeping your back straight.

Take a firm grip on the rope and if needed loop it around your hands. In that position, using your lower back muscles and glutes as the primary drivers, lift into a deadlift position to perform the exercise.

When you perform an isometric exercise never hold your breath. Always breathe deeply and naturally, which will be about 10 full breaths at a rate of about 1 second per breath.

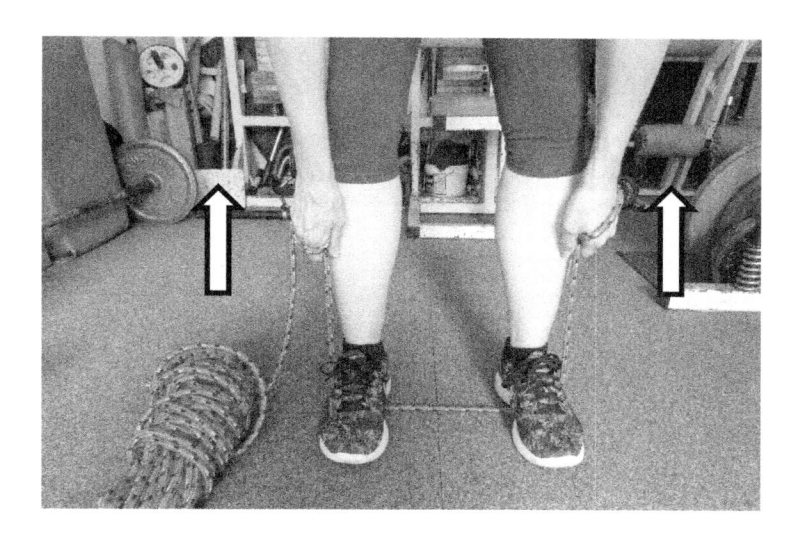

Perform each exercise for no less than 7 seconds, and no longer than 10.

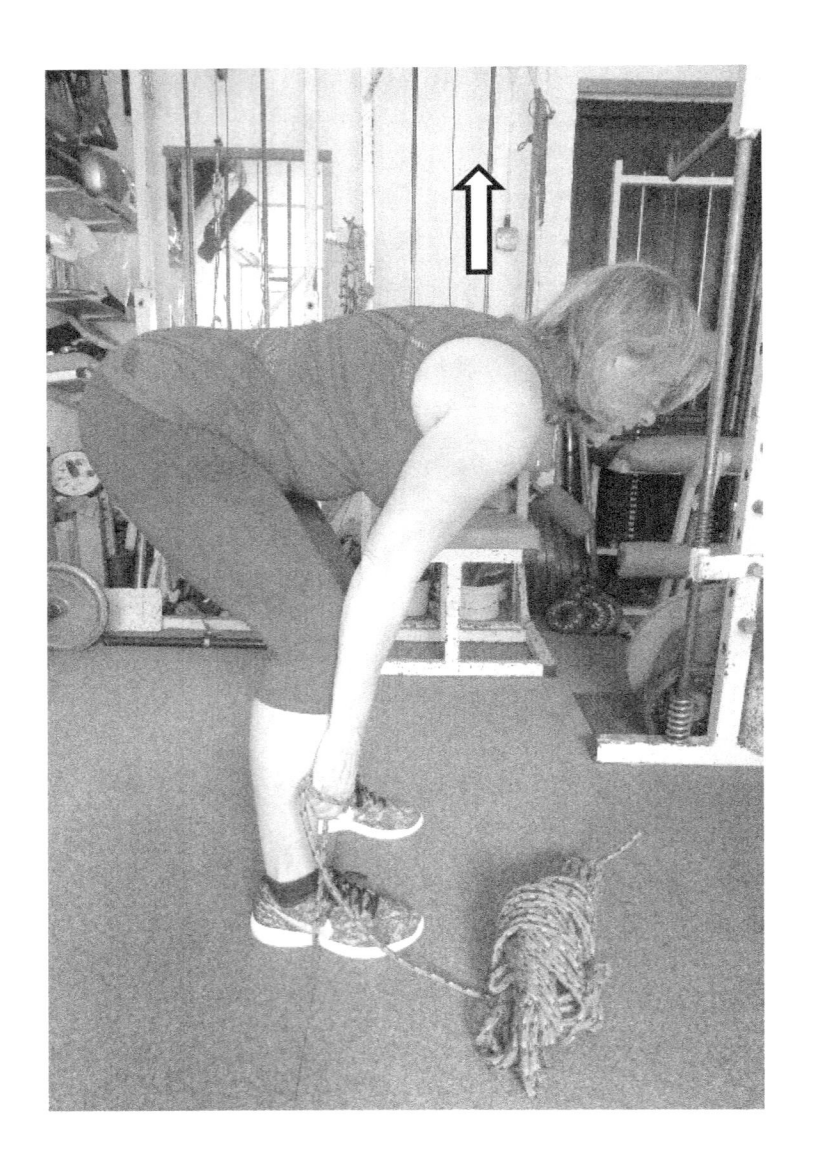

6) Chest: Palm-Press Together

In either a seated or standing position, bring the palms of your hands together in front of your chest.

Ensure that your elbows and arms are out and to the side, so your upper arms are approximately parallel to the floor.

In this position, using the chest muscles as the primary drivers, press your hands together to perform the exercise.

When you perform an isometric exercise never hold your breath. Always breathe deeply and naturally, which will be about 10 full breaths at a rate of about 1 second per breath.

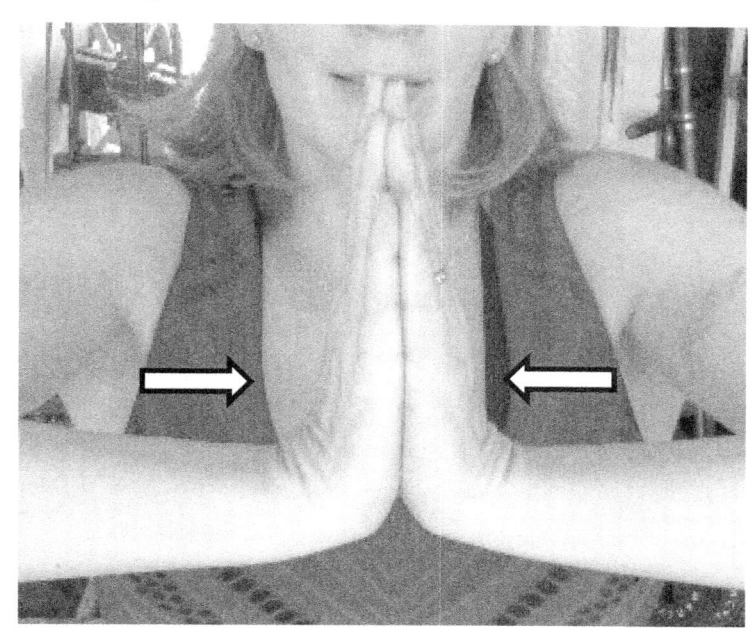

Perform each exercise for no less than 7 seconds, and no longer than 10.

111

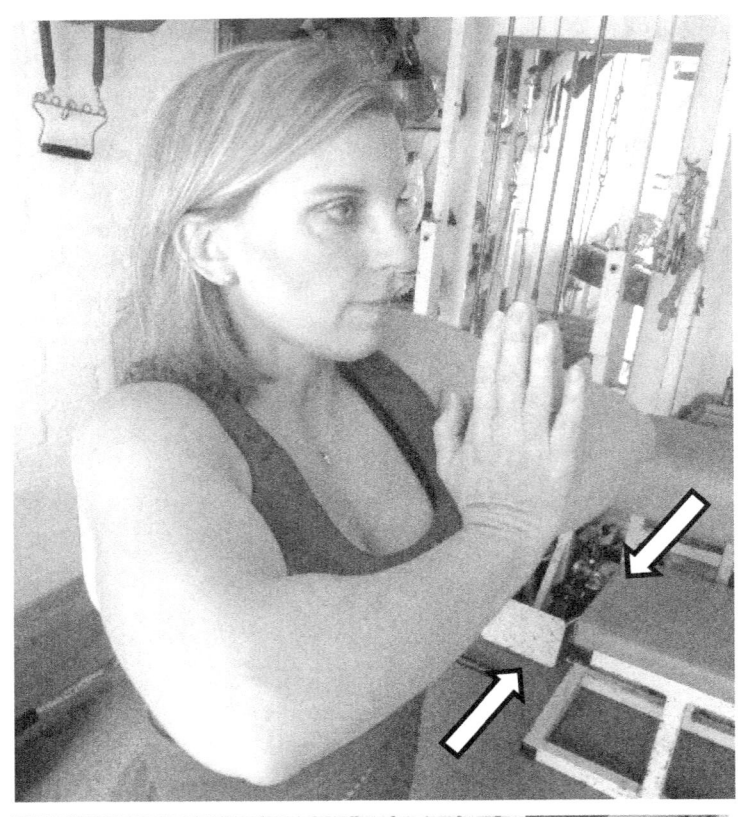

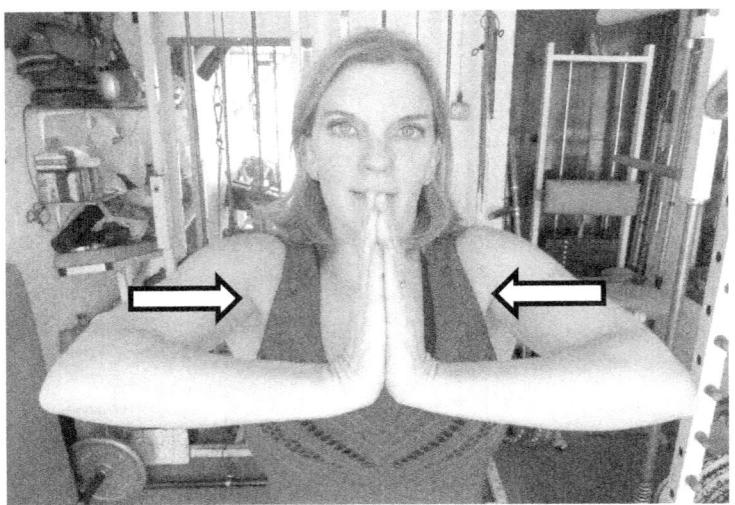

Variation Chest: Press Together with Rope Looped Around Hands

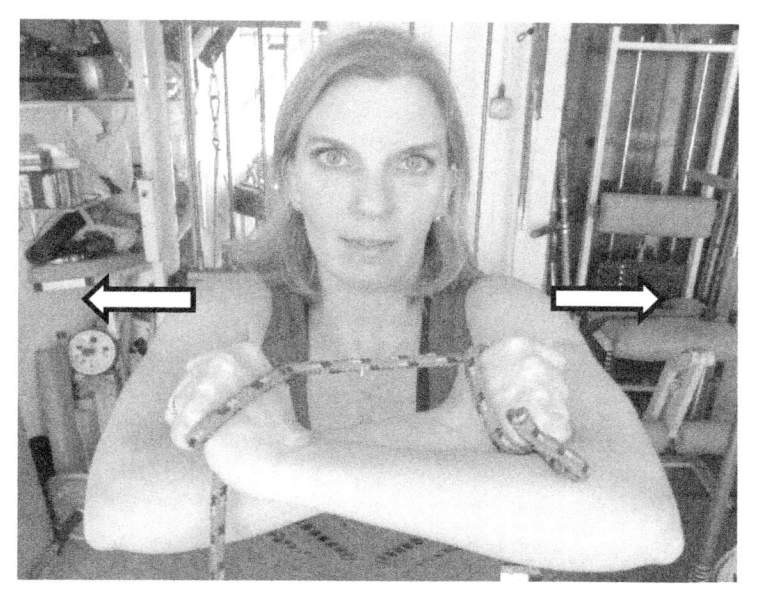

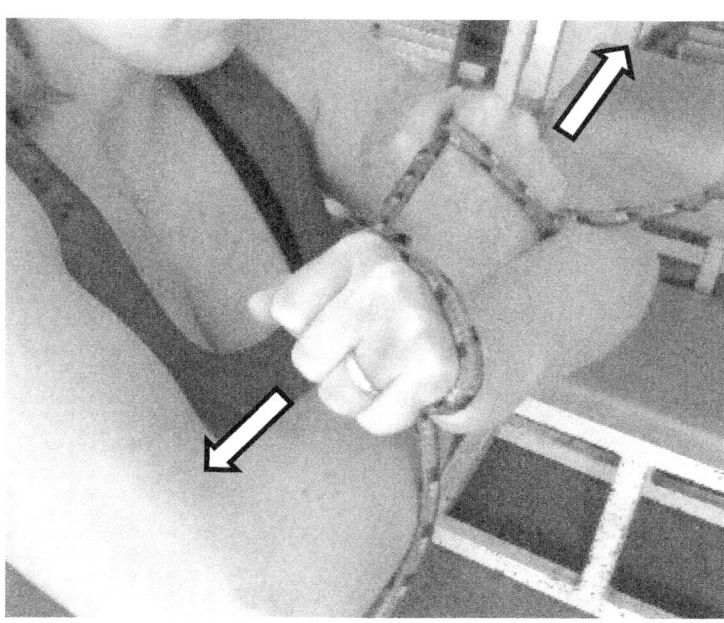

Variation Chest: Press Together with Iso-Bow®

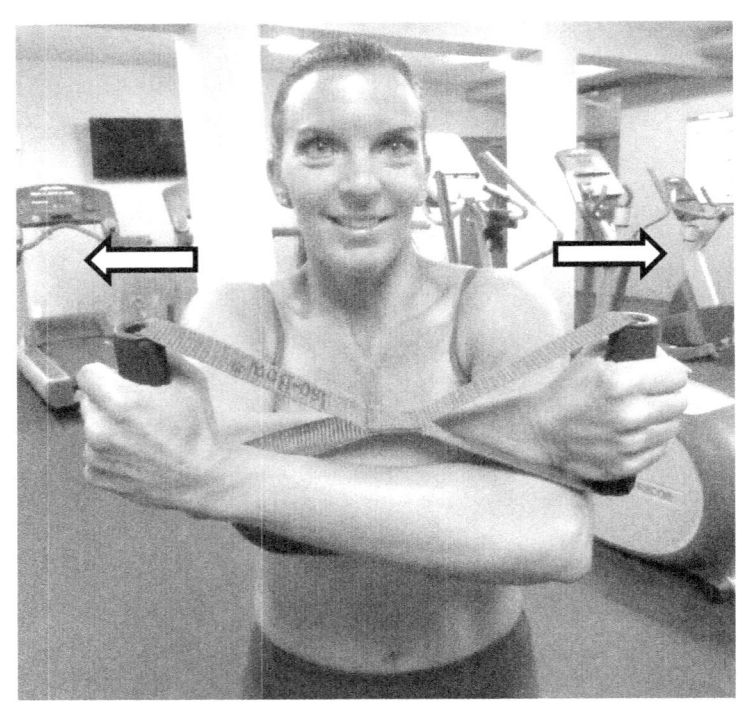

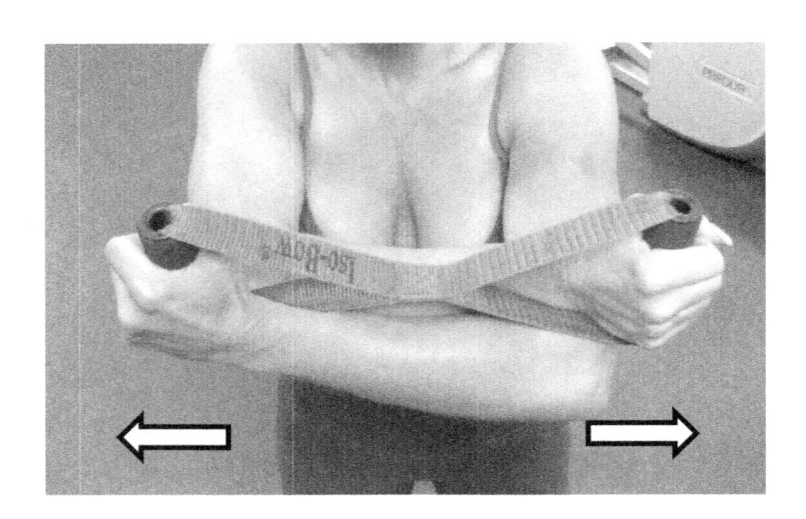

7) Shoulders: Side Lateral Raise Hands Interlock

Stand upright and interlock your fingers and hands in front of you at arm's length. Bend both arms slightly in a no-lock elbow position.

Attempt to raise the arms sideways using your shoulder muscles as the driving force to perform the deltoid exercise.

When you perform an isometric exercise never hold your breath. Always breathe deeply and naturally, which will be about 10 full breaths at a rate of about 1 second per breath.

Perform each exercise for no less than 7 seconds, and no longer than 10.

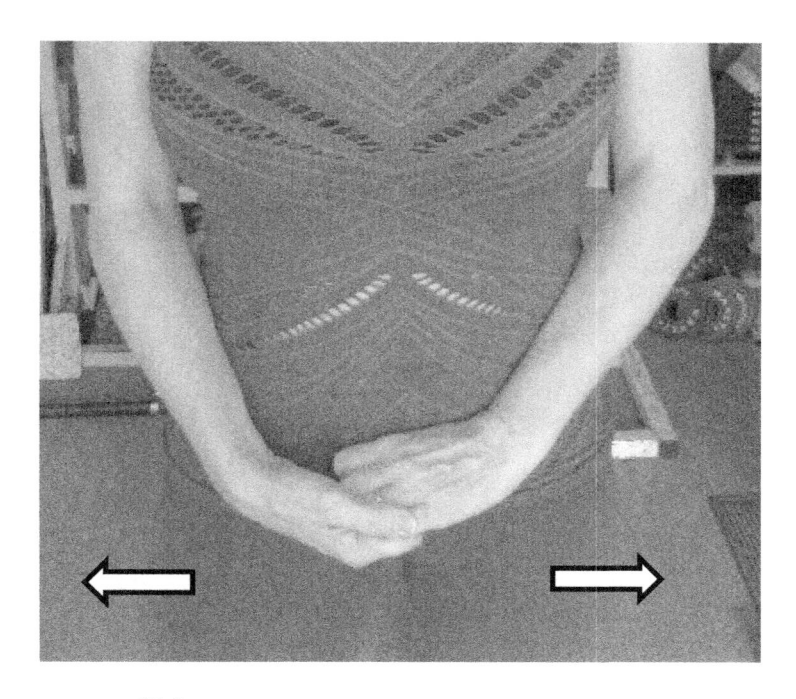

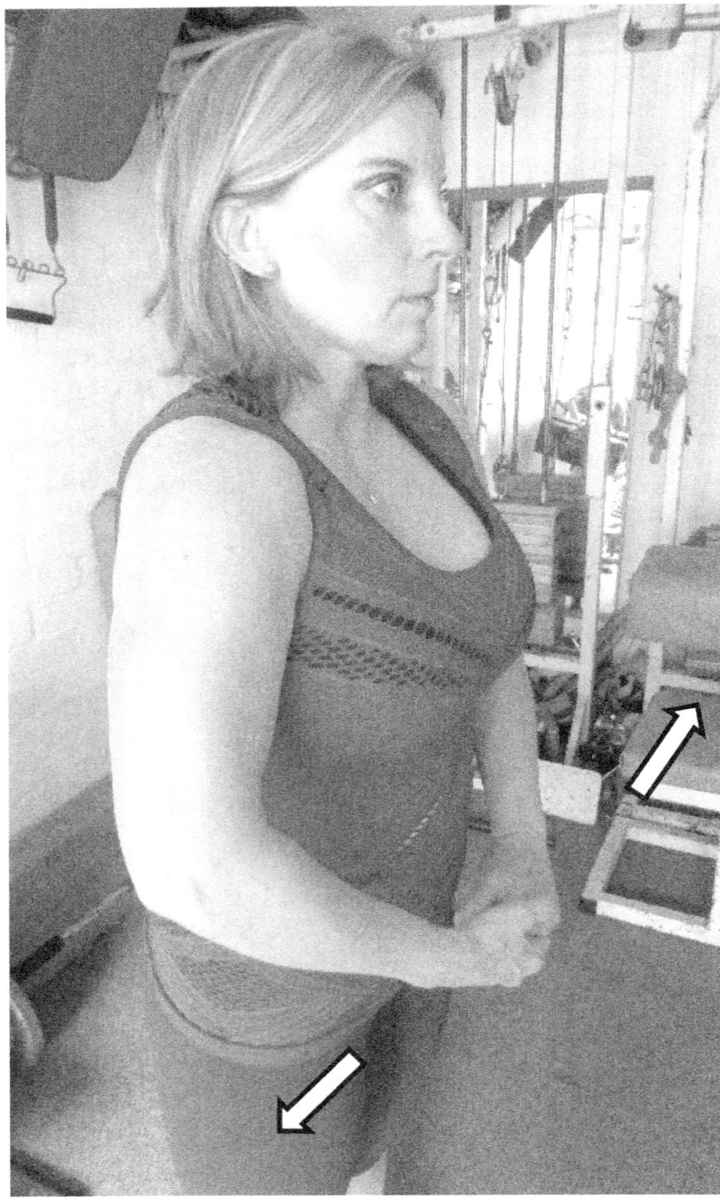

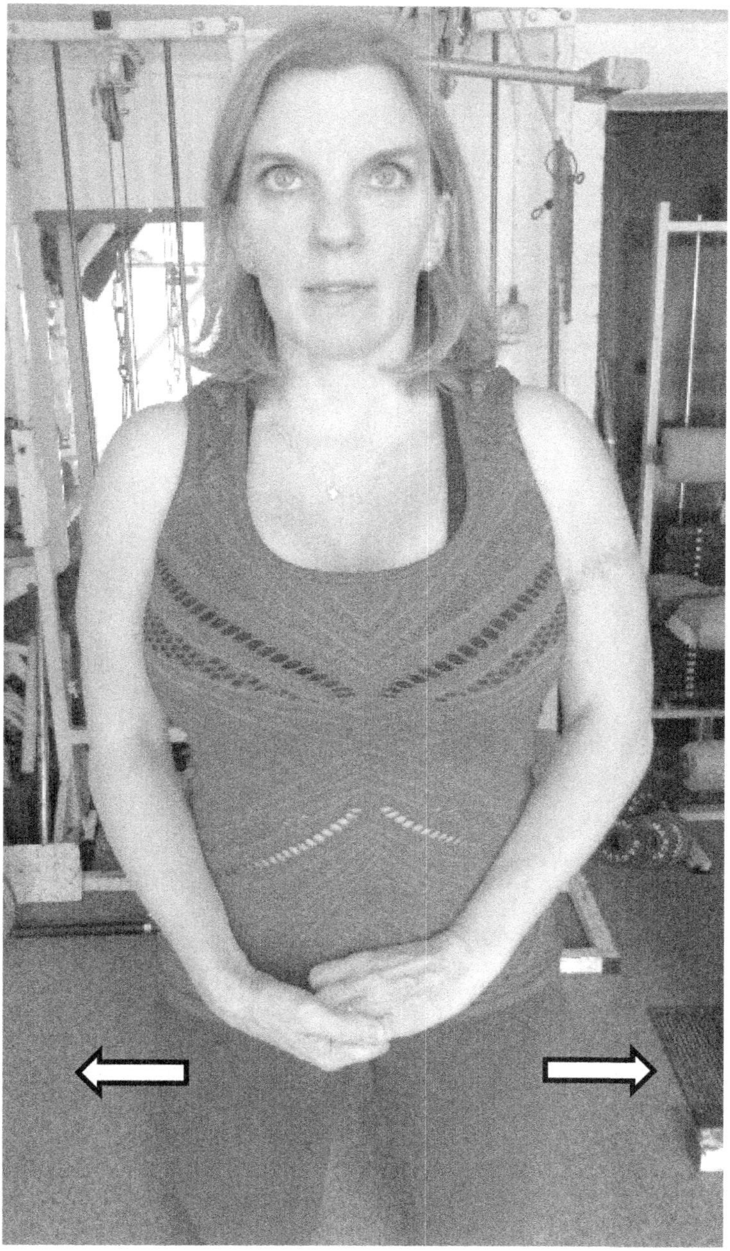

Variation Shoulders:
Side Lateral Raise with Rope

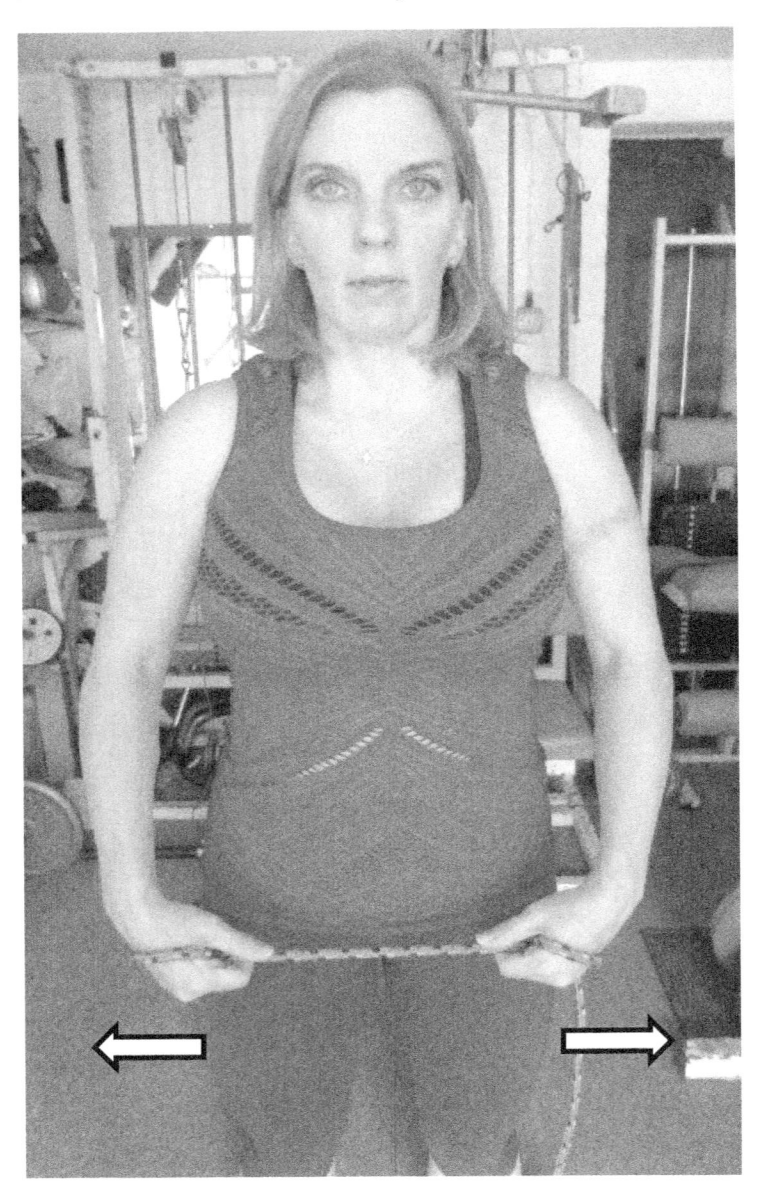

Variation Shoulders:
Side Lateral Raise with Towel

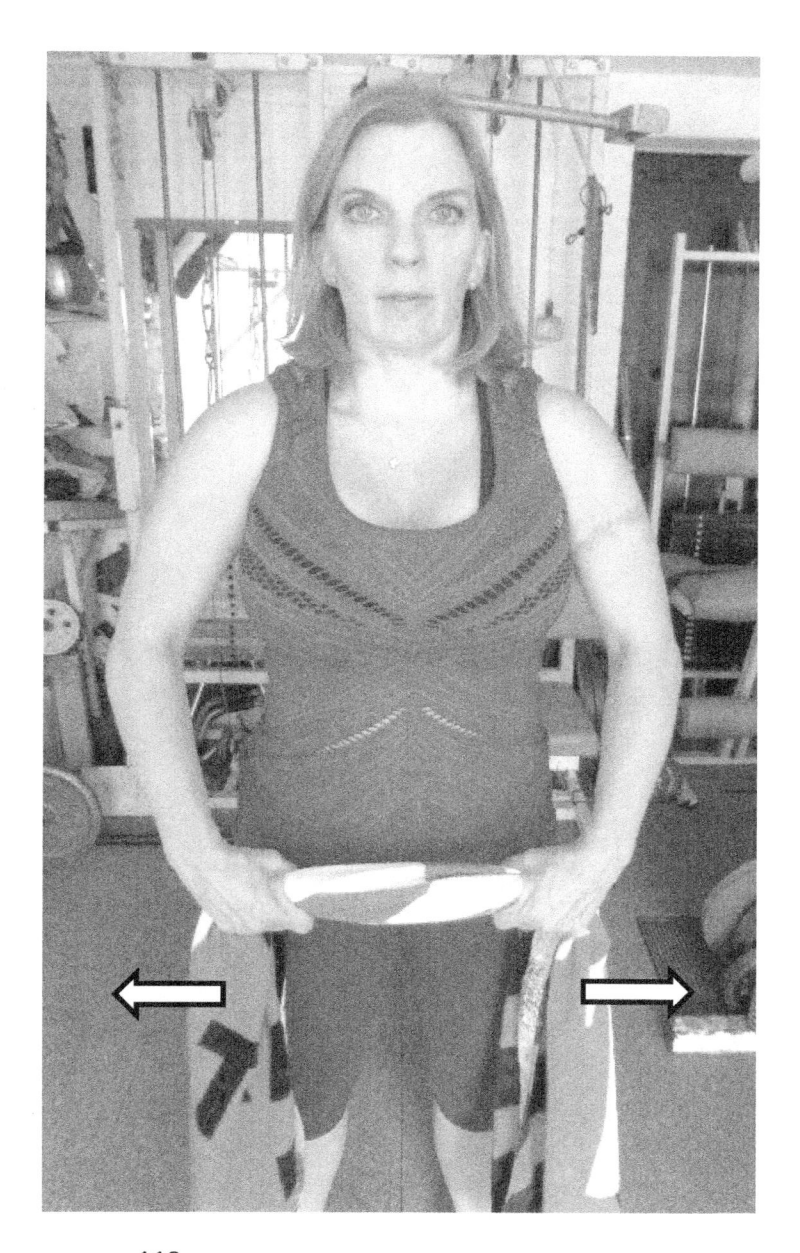

Variation Shoulders:
Side Lateral Raise with Iso-Bow®

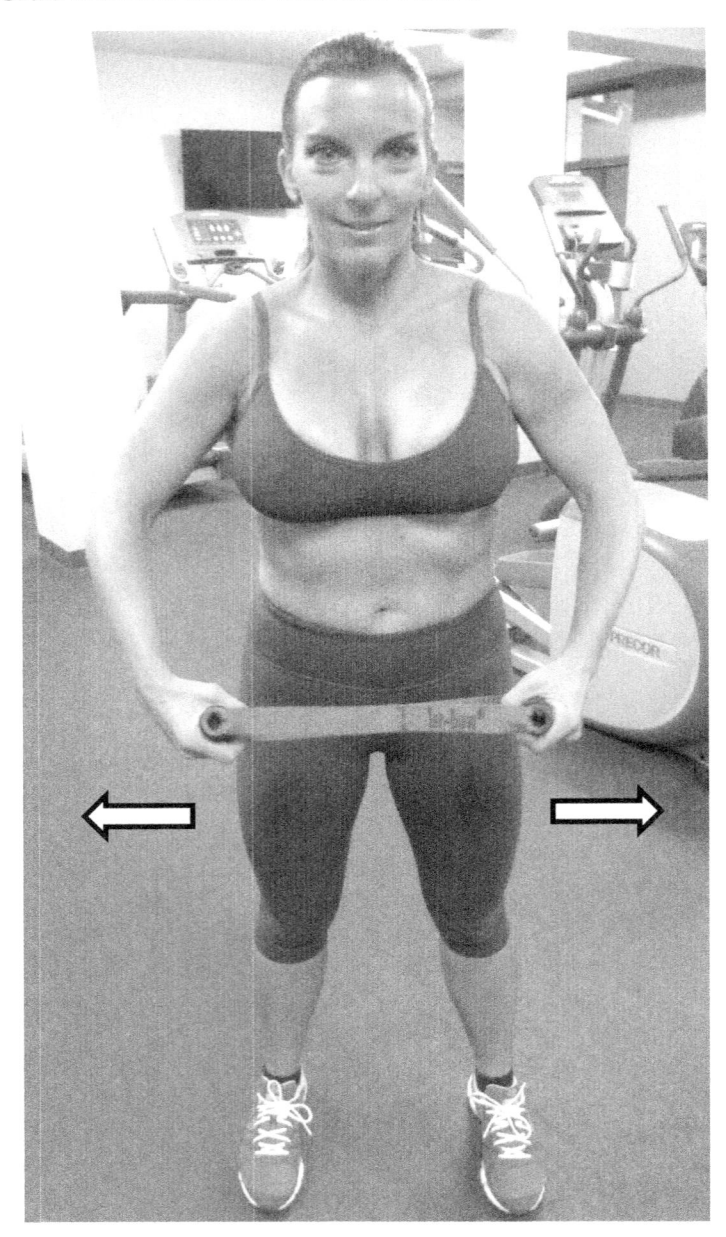

Variation Shoulders:
Side Lateral Raise with Rope Under Feet

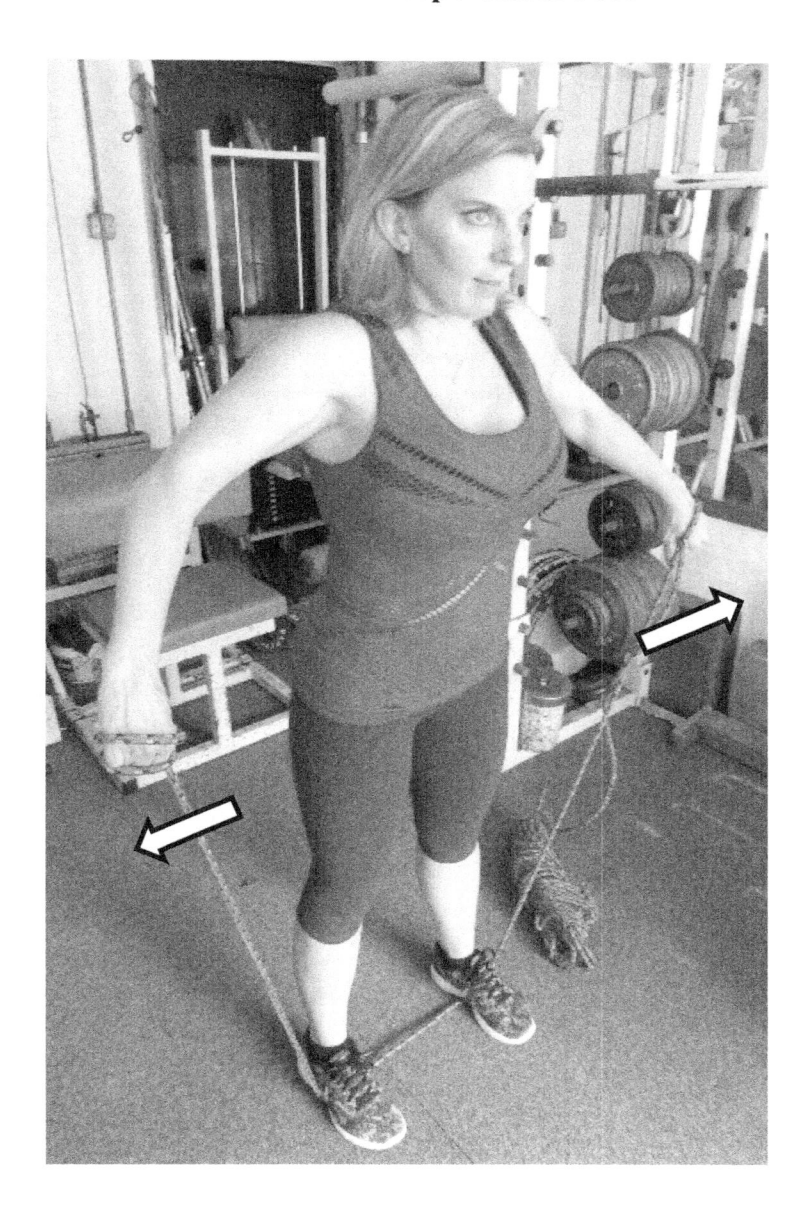

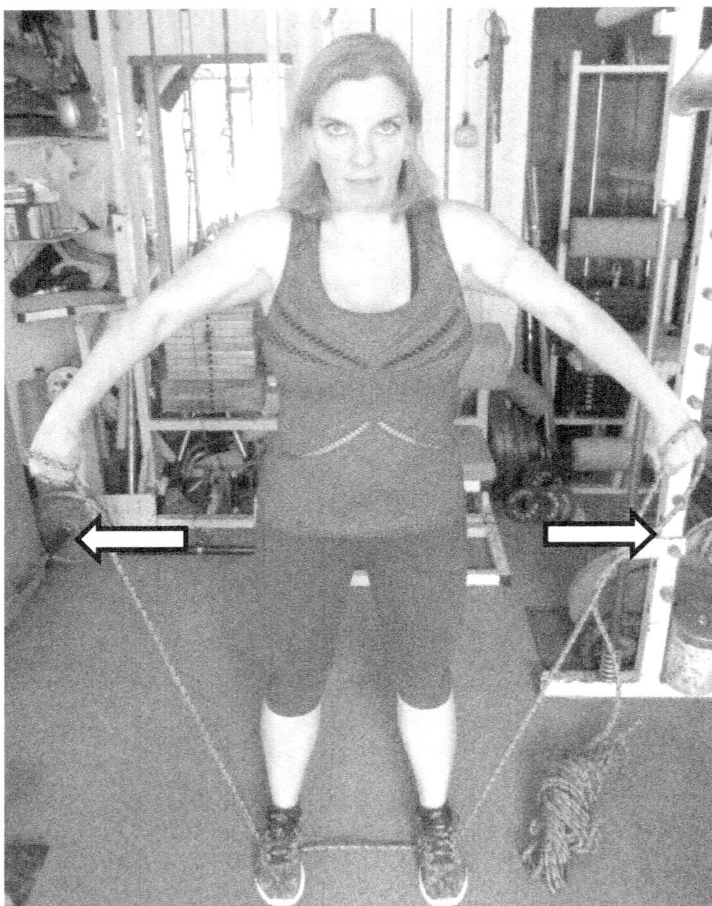

8) Upper Thighs Front: Wall Squat

Stand with your feet approximately shoulder-width apart slightly away from a solid wall or door that will not open.

Squat down with your thighs approximately parallel to the floor while leaning against the wall/door with your entire torso and glutes.

Pushing backwards and slightly upwards, attempt to stand up from the squat lower position to engage the thighs and glutes to perform the exercise.

When you perform an isometric exercise never hold your breath. Always breathe deeply and naturally, which will be about 10 full breaths at a rate of about 1 second per breath.

Perform each exercise for no less than 7 seconds, and no longer than 10.

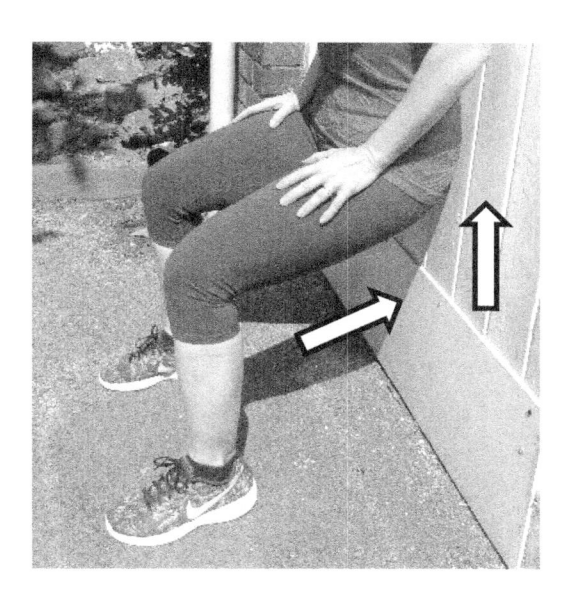

123

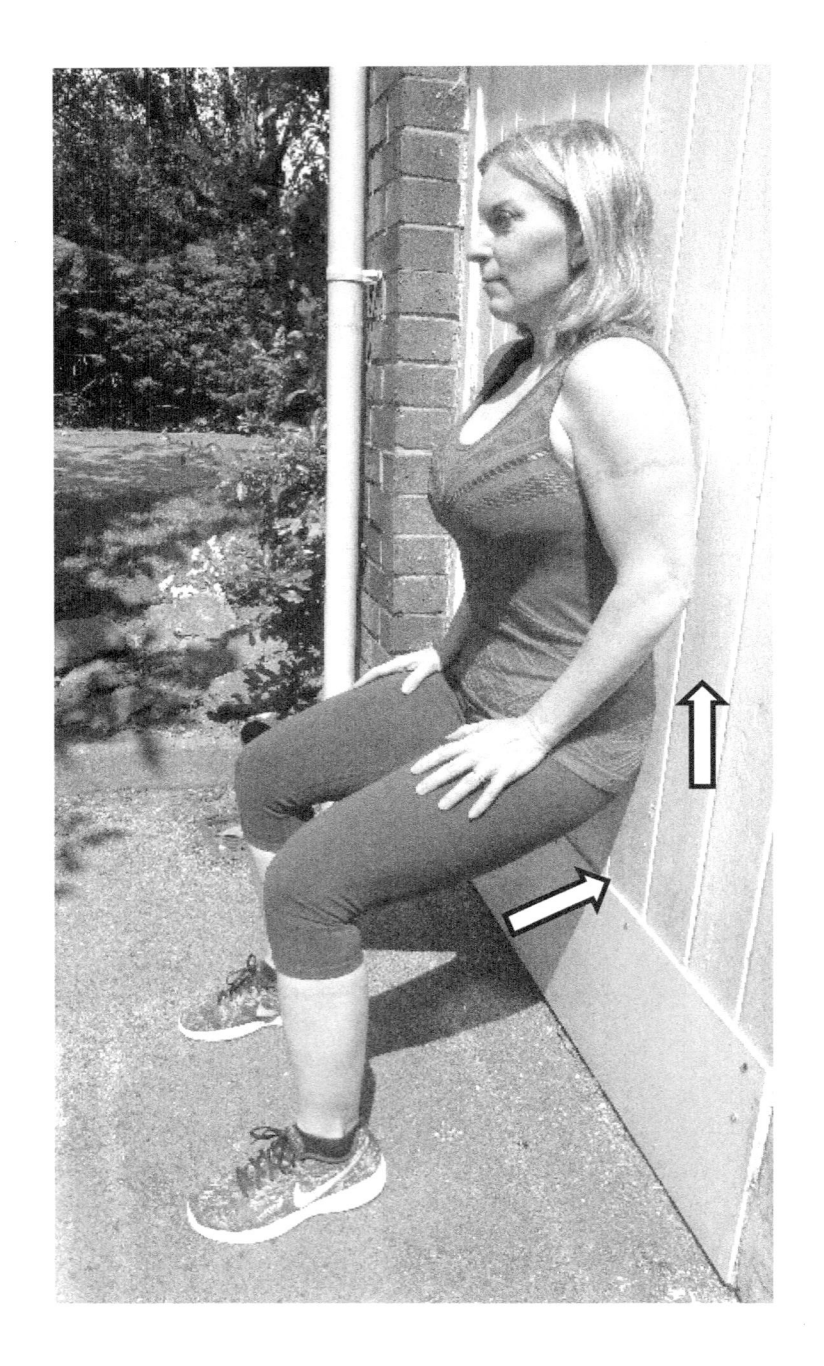

Variation Upper Thighs Front: Squat with Rope

Stand with your feet approximately shoulder-width apart on a suitable length of strong rope which is positioned well under both feet.

Squat down by bending the knees and torso by bending only from the hip to keep the back straight.

Holding the rope securely in each hand at an appropriate position, attempt to stand up from the squat lower position to engage the thighs and glutes to perform the exercise.

When you perform an isometric exercise never hold your breath. Always breathe deeply and naturally, which will be about 10 full breaths at a rate of about 1 second per breath.

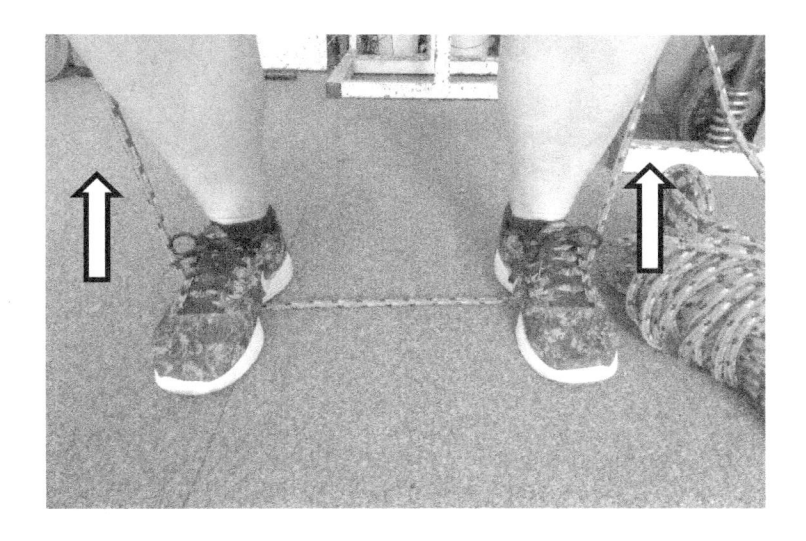

Perform each exercise for no less than 7 seconds, and no longer than 10.

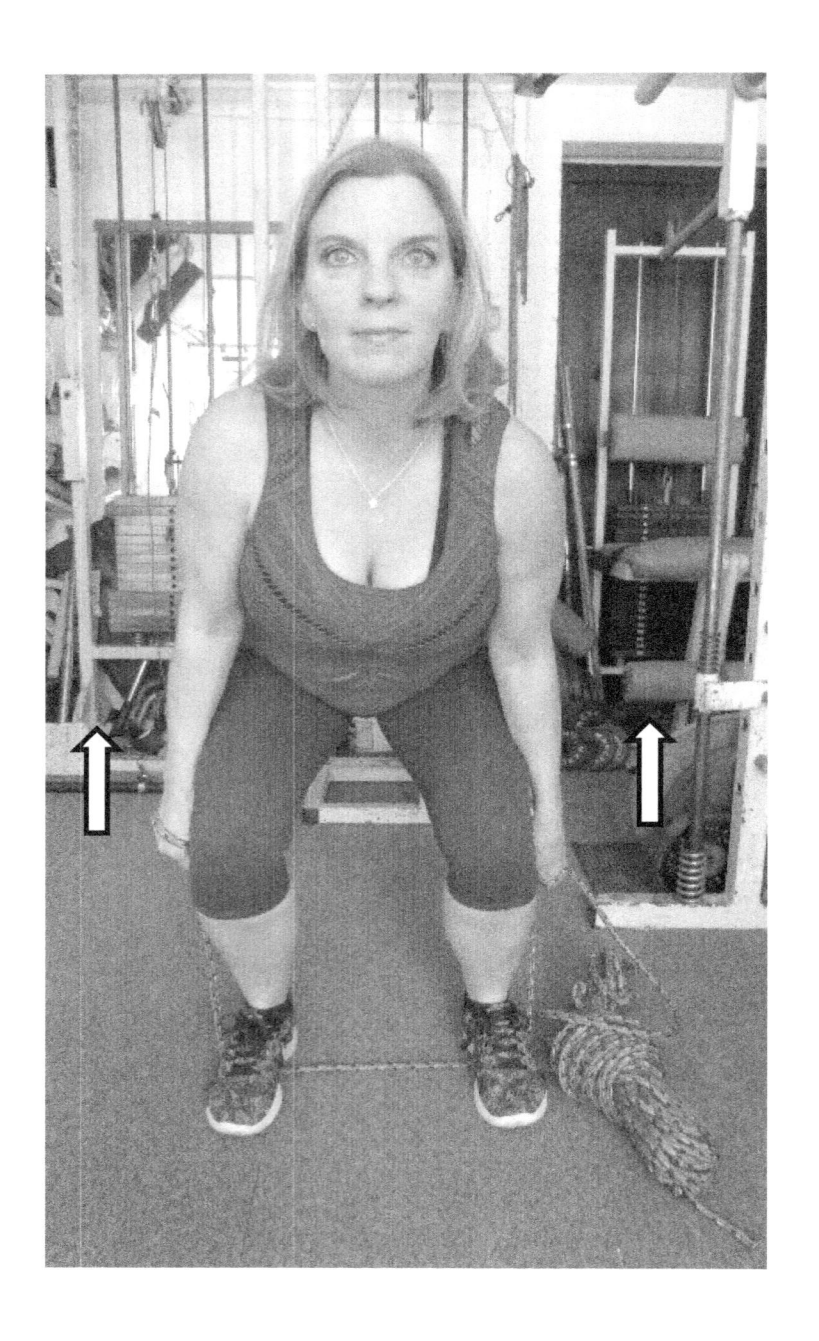

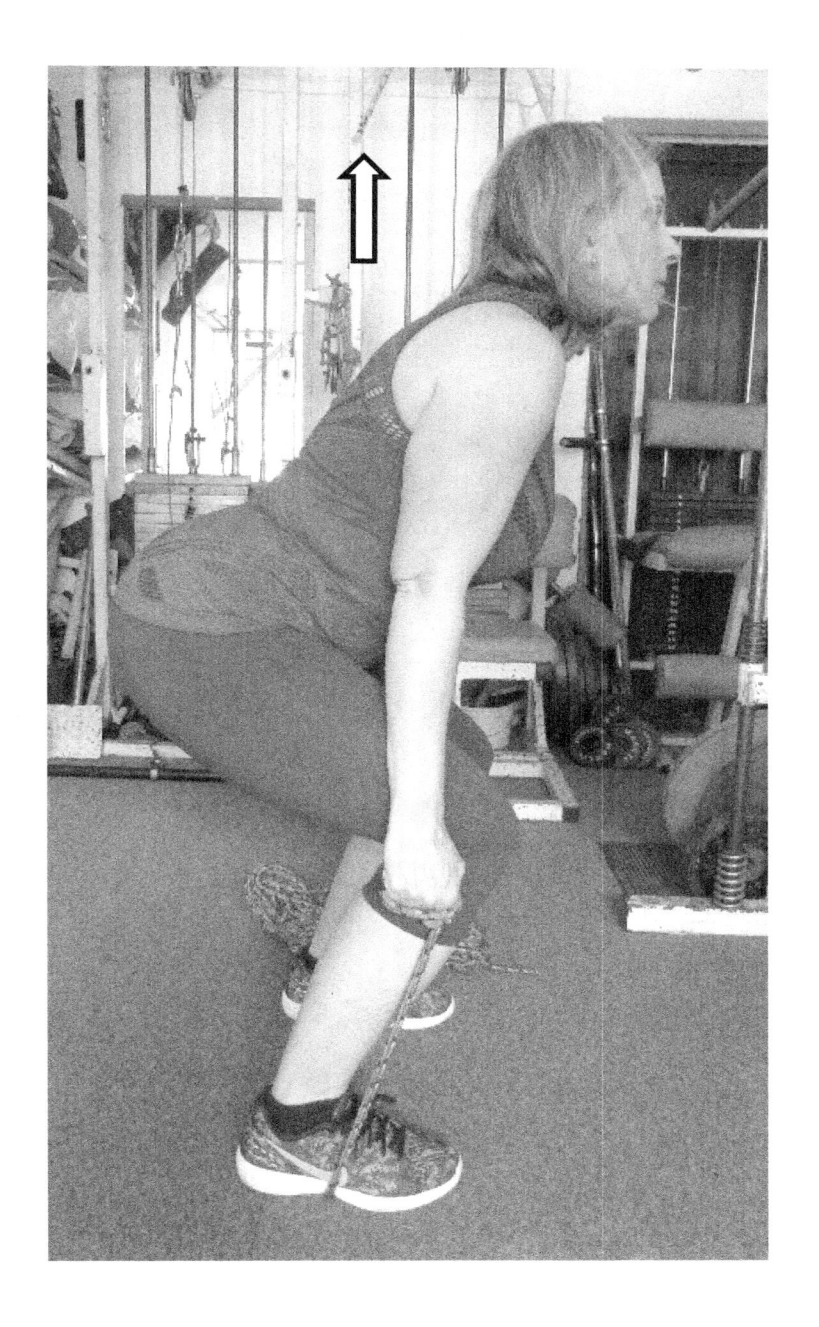

9) Upper Thigh Hamstring: Wall Hamstring Curl

To perform the wall hamstring curl, stand with your feet slightly away from a wall or other solid object. In this position, raise one leg slightly to the rear so that the heel meets the wall/object.

Keep your foot and toes pulled up and toward your knee at all times. With your back flat against the wall, attempt to curl your leg by pushing the heel into the wall and upwards to perform the exercise. Do not forget the other leg.

When you perform an isometric exercise never hold your breath. Always breathe deeply and naturally, which will be about 10 full breaths at a rate of about 1 second per breath.

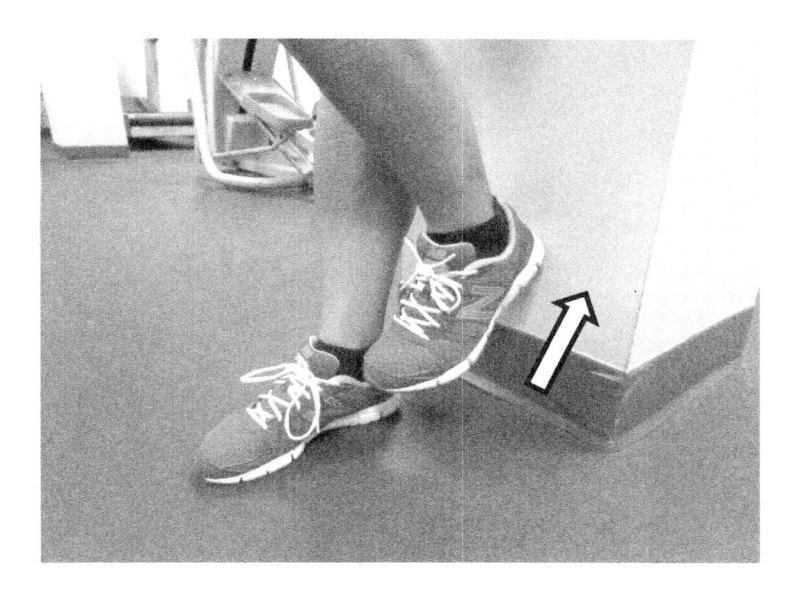

Perform each exercise for no less than 7 seconds, and no longer than 10.

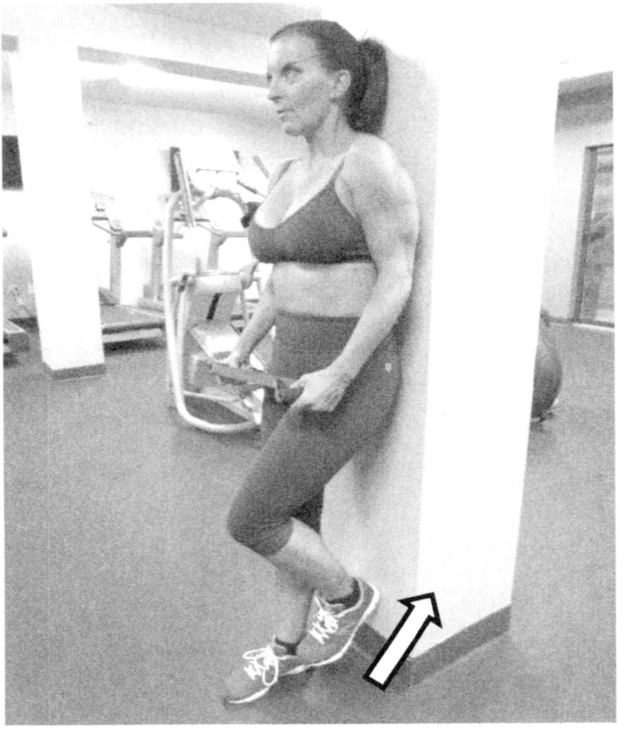

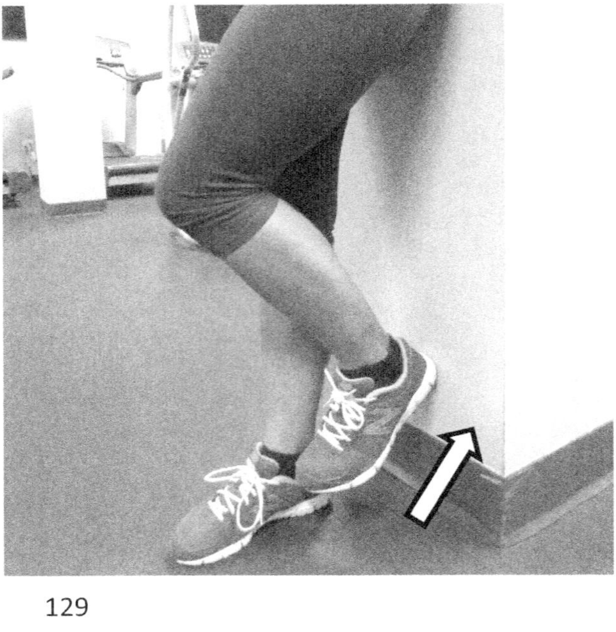

10) Calf: Immovable Object Heel Raise-Push

Stand in front of a wall or any other solid immovable object at arm's length from you as you place the palms of your hands on it.

Step backwards with one leg and place your foot flat on the floor behind you. In this position, use the calf muscles of the rear foot as the driver.

Push as you attempt to raise the heel of your foot as you attempt to move the immovable object to perform the exercise.

When you perform an isometric exercise never hold your breath. Always breathe deeply and naturally, which will be about 10 full breaths at a rate of about 1 second per breath. Perform each exercise for no less than 7 seconds, and no longer than 10. Do not forget to exercise both legs.

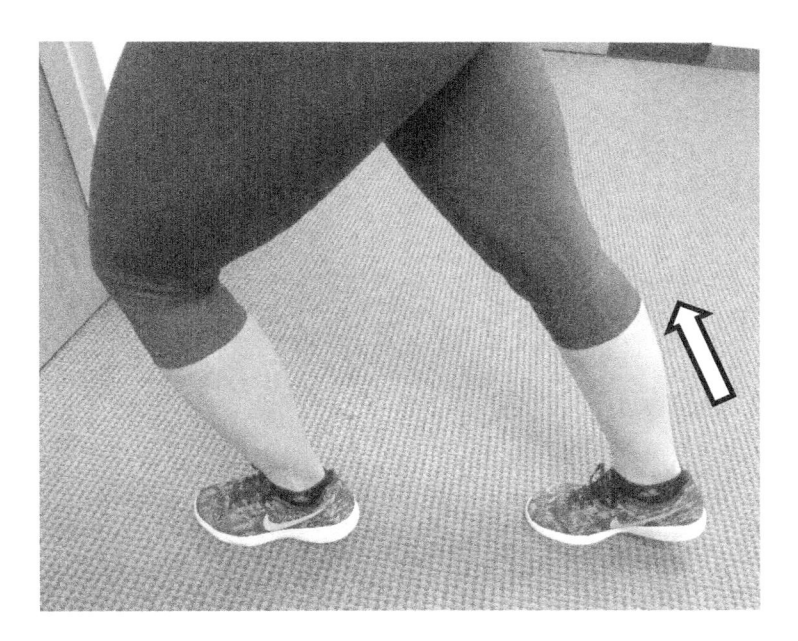

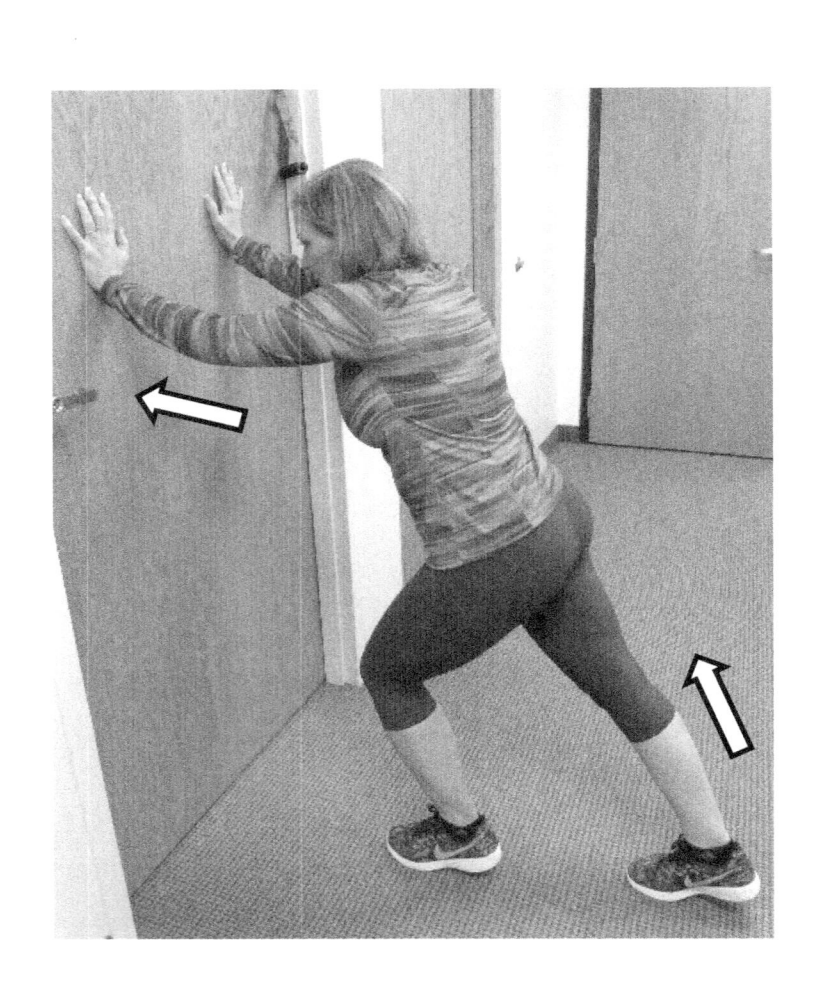

Chapter 7: Conclusion

We sincerely hope that you decide to take the physical action of trying The 70 Second Difference™ protocol. It is possibly the shortest workout possible that will exercise all the major muscles of the body with as much or little intensity you choose to apply. The choice is always yours, the more effort and intensity you put in to teach exercise, the greater the benefits that you will receive from the exercise routine.

The 10 exercises of The 70 Second Difference™ protocol obviously takes 70 seconds of consecutive exercise time to perform. However, with a 10 to 20-second rest between exercises, or longer, this can increase the overall workout time to around 5 minutes. However, this is still an exceptionally short time spent exercising, especially when one considers the comparative times. If the workout takes 5 minutes to perform with extended rest times between exercises, only 70 seconds of that overall time is actually spent performing exercises.

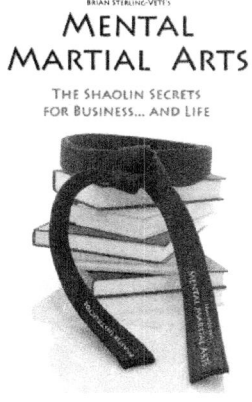

You may also wish to explore some of the techniques I wrote about in the book Mental Martial Arts. As a martial arts instructor, the approach I take to life, business and motivational strategy and tactics are based on the teachings of several different styles of the martial arts. Many have found that this approach makes the concepts easier to understand and apply in practice to everyday real-world scenarios. My system of Mental Martial Arts has been used in this way by many companies and government organisations including Eli Lilly Pharmaceuticals and ST. Paul Public School District.

Feed your mind with positive thoughts every day. This is similar to how we physically feed our physical body with food to fuel us each day. If the foods we consume are high-quality healthy foods, then this will typically lead to us having a healthier body with fewer physical problems. If the foods are low-quality junk-type foods, then we should not be surprised when we become sick, develop health issues and function poorly. This is simply basic common sense because we are what we eat.

The same is true of our mental health because we are what we think. Therefore, we need to feed our mind every day with positive, emotionally nutritious thoughts and feelings. If you do something for at least 21 days, then it psychologists tell us that it becomes a habit, and in this case, one which is good for us.

Another great way to do this is to listen to motivational recordings. Any will do, the choice is yours. If you find some that you particularly enjoy then that is fantastic because you should look forward to your daily food for thought every bit as much as looking forward to enjoying the food you eat for your body.

We highly recommend the recordings and seminars of my old friend Zig Ziglar. Zig is not just motivational and inspirational; he has also got a great sense of humour too.

Even though I now know many of his seminars and recordings by heart, they still make me laugh aloud, which in and of itself is great uplifting medicine. Also, Zig has thoroughly researched the subject and has worked with some of the finest specialists in the world. This means that his seminars and recordings are packed with interesting and valuable resources and information. Take a look at them for yourself at https://www.ziglar.com/

You may also wish to read some of the excellent research studies that have been performed about how exercise can help to treat and beat depression. Here are some you may wish to search for online to read.

- Is Exercise a Viable Treatment for Depression? By James A. Blumenthal, Ph.D., Patrick J. Smith, Ph.D., and Benson M. Hoffman, Ph.D.
- Exercise and the Prevention of Depression: Results of the HUNT Cohort Study by Samuel B. Harvey, F.R.A.N.Z.C.P., Ph.D., Simon Øverland, Ph.D., Stephani L. Hatch, Ph.D., Simon Wessely, F.R.C.Psych., M.D., Arnstein Mykletun, Ph.D., Matthew Hotopf, F.R.C.Psych., Ph.D.
- Physical Activity and Exercise in the Treatment of Depression by Professor Holly Blake, Associate Professor of Behavioural Science, Faculty of Medicine & Health Sciences University of Nottingham https://www.nottingham.ac.uk/healthsciences/people/holly.blake

We now urge you to remember the words of my friend, the great Zig Ziglar and "Logic will not change a feeling or emotion, only a physical action will." Take the physical action of following The 70 Second Difference™ protocol every day for a month. We are certain that you will both see a difference physically and feel a difference emotionally too. We sincerely believe that you can begin to feel better in just 70 seconds, so give it a try.

We wish you luck, good health, and to feel good about yourself and your life. You are unique, a special person who makes the world an infinitely better place because you are here. For more information about isometric exercise and the online video resources for TWiEA members, visit www.TWiEA.com

What is TWiEA™?

TWiEA™ is the acronym for The World Isometric Exercise Association which is the global governing body for all types of isometric exercise. TWiEA™'s mission is to help set and maintain standards of excellence in teaching and promoting all types of isometric exercise. TWiEA™'s mission is to ensure that scientifically proven time-efficient isometric exercise techniques are taught to clients as part of an integrated overall approach to the total-body exercise solutions provided by fitness professionals. This creates a much higher probability that clients who are busy people, and who often face real-life time-crunches, can still maintain a regular highly effective exercise program. The fact is that isometric exercise is every bit as effective, and frequently more effective, at building muscle and strength as other more traditional forms of resistance training. It is also a timesaving and money-saving exercise solution that almost anyone can perform, even without equipment.

www.MajorVision.com

Other books by Brian Sterling-Vete and Helen Renée Wuorio

The 70 Second Difference™ - The Politically Incorrect, Occasionally Amusing, and Brutally Effective Guide to Strength, Fitness and Better Health

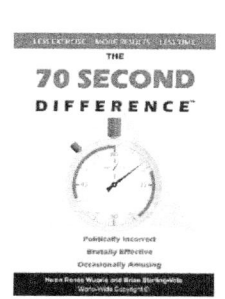

This book has been approved by **TWiEA** – The World Isometric Exercise Association (www.TWiEA.com).

This is a science-based no-nonsense guide that tells it straight about the most efficient ways to exercise, build muscle, get strong and how your deliberate lifestyle choices directly affect your body weight, overall health, fitness, strength, and body shape. It also tells you how much protein you really need, and the dangers associated with dairy and animal-based products and meat. Lack of time is typically the enemy of fitness and regular exercise routines, however, just 70 seconds a day of focussed science-based exercise can solve the problem. Recommended equipment: 2 x Iso-Bows®

The ISOmetric Bible™ - Exercise Anywhere with Scientifically Proven Isometrics

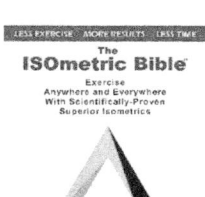

This book has been approved by **TWiEA** – The World Isometric Exercise Association (www.TWiEA.com).

At 330+ pages, the ISOmetric Bible™ is one of the most complete, scientific, practical, and user-friendly books on isometrics that has ever been written. Isometrics are proven by science to grow muscle and strength faster and more efficiently than any other exercise system. However, isometrics are also one of the most misunderstood forms of exercise, even by fitness professionals. An isometric exercise routine takes only minutes each day and can be performed anywhere you choose, on a plane, in a car, or even while you are at work. You do not need any special equipment to get a great total-body workout and the book shows you how to use easy to find everyday objects such as walking poles, broom handles, rope, and towels to exercise with. Recommended equipment: 2 x Iso-Bows®, some climbing rope and a towel.

Workout at Work™ - Exercise at Work Without Anyone Even Knowing What You're Doing!

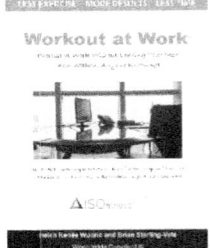

This book has been approved by **TWiEA** – The World Isometric Exercise Association (www.TWiEA.com).

Time is the #1 reason why people do not exercise. The average person spends over 10 years of their life at work over an average 45 year working life, which can mean sitting at a desk for 10-years! With proven isometric exercise, you can exercise so effectively at work that even a complete beginner can benefit as much as an advanced athlete without ever leaving your desk. Just one simple 7-second high-intensity exercise every 30 minutes at your desk and at the end of a 9-hour working day you will have completed a powerful total-body 18-20 exercise. Your boss will not complain either because in exchange for just 126 seconds of time off work you will be up to 30% more efficient at your job. Required equipment: 2 x Iso-Bows® available on Amazon or from Bullworker.com

TRISOmetrics™ - Advanced Science-Based High-Intensity Strength and Muscle Building

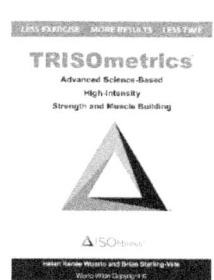

This book has been approved by **TWiEA** – The World Isometric Exercise Association (www.TWiEA.com).

TRISOmetrics™ is an advanced, science-based high-intensity exercise system which combines 3 scientifically proven exercise techniques into a powerful new exercise system. It can be performed with or without equipment either at home or when travelling, or it can be used as part of a gym-based exercise routine. It focusses on precision and quality in each exercise combined with high-intensity to engage the maximum number of muscle fibres which keeps exercise sessions short, infrequent, and highly effective. The system is ideal for people who do not confuse activity with accomplishment. Suggested equipment: 2 x Iso-Bows®, climbing rope and a towel. It can also be performed with the Bullworker®, Steel Bow®, Bow Extension®, Iso-Gym® or similar and with all gym-based exercise equipment.

The TRISO90™ Course – Advanced Strength and Muscle Building with The TRISOmetrics™ System

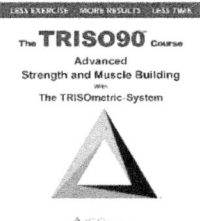

This book has been approved by **TWiEA** – The World Isometric Exercise Association (www.TWiEA.com).

The TRISO90™ Course is a 500+ page 90-day/12-week step-by-step highly advanced bodybuilding and strength-training exercise course based on the TRISOmetrics™

exercise system. The system consists of three proven science-based exercise principles which when combined, form this highly advanced high-intensity exercise technique. This is a highly advanced pure strength and muscle building ideal for the natural bodybuilder or for anyone who wants to get into the best shape possible in the minimum amount of time, with or without equipment. Suggested equipment: 2 x Iso-Bows®, dipping handles, some climbing rope, and a towel.

Isometric Power Exercises for Martial Arts™ - Build Superior Strength, Muscle and Martial Arts 'Firepower' Using the Proven System Bruce Lee Used

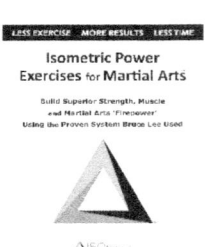

This book has been approved by **TWiEA** – The World Isometric Exercise Association (www.TWiEA.com).

Isometric exercise is a part of almost every system of the martial arts. Even before isometrics were studied scientifically, isometrics were taught and practised in one form or another for thousands of years. More recently, it was the great Bruce Lee and his love of isometric exercise who ensured that they would become famously linked to all types of martial arts training. This book is a valuable resource of practical isometric exercises to build serious strength, muscle and martial arts 'firepower' needed by all types of martial artists. They build solid, hard, practical muscle and not the bodybuilder type of bulk that would seriously restrict a martial artist. The author is recognised as one of the leading authorities on isometric exercise and has practised several different styles of martial arts for almost 50-years. Among his many awards and accolades, he is a WKA 8th Degree Black Belt and a recipient of a WKA Lifetime Achievement Award.

Fitness on the Move™ - Enjoy Gym-Quality Workout Sessions ANYWHERE!

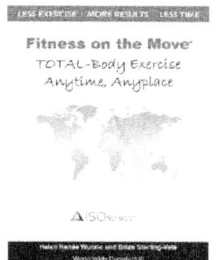

This book has been approved by **TWiEA** – The World Isometric Exercise Association (www.TWiEA.com).

Both beginners and professional athletes alike can maintain a great workout routine while travelling away from home and the gym. The Fitness on the Move™ book is a list of exercises that can deliver a full-body workout in the smallest space humanly possible thanks to our Zero Footprint Workout™ concept. If there is enough space to either sit down or stand upright, then you can perform a total-body exercise routine. We have tested the Fitness on the Move™ system as passengers in cars, on trains, in airline seats, on mountainsides, on beaches, and once even on the deck of a ship in a storm. Required/suggested equipment: 2 x Iso-Bows® available on Amazon or from Bullworker.com

The ISO90™ Course – The 12-Week/90-Day Shape-up and Get Strong Course

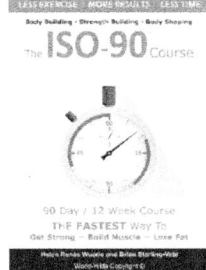

This book has been approved by **TWiEA** – The World Isometric Exercise Association (www.TWiEA.com).

The ISO90™ Course is a comprehensive and complete step by step 90-day/12-week step-by-step isometric body shaping, bodybuilding, and functional strength building course. It is ideal for both beginners and advanced trainers because your natural Adaptive Response™ mechanism means that whatever intensity you apply at whatever level you are gives everyone roughly the same percentage of improvement. Required equipment: 2 x Iso-Bows® available on Amazon or from Bullworker.com

The Bullworker Bible™ The Ultimate Science-Based Guide to The Classic Personal Multi-Gym

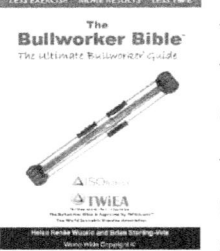

This book has been approved by **TWiEA** – The World Isometric Exercise Association (www.TWiEA.com).

The Bullworker Bible™ is the definitive resource guide for all Bullworker® users, and it is the companion book for The Bullworker 90™ Course and is approved by the makers of The Bullworker. It is a complete science-based user-friendly guide of how the Bullworker® should be used properly to deliver maximum results. It gives you all the information about repetition-compression and speed control, correct breathing techniques, how Hooke's Law of physics applies to The Bullworker®, and about correct biomechanics to deliver the best results. The Bullworker Bible™ is also the essential guide for all users of the Steel Bow®, Bullworker X5, Bully Extreme, ISO 7x, and the Bullworker X7. Required equipment: Bullworker® Classic, or similar. Recommended additional equipment: Steel Bow®, 2 x Iso-Bows®, and Bow Extension®.

The Bullworker 90™ Course – The Ultimate Science-Based 12-Week/90-Day Get strong and Grow Muscle Course Using the Classic Personal Multi-Gym

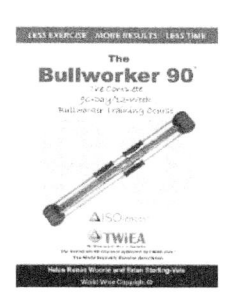

This book has been approved by **TWiEA** – The World Isometric Exercise Association (www.TWiEA.com).

The Bullworker 90™ Course is a 400+ page 90-day/12-week step-by-step course for all Bullworker® users and the companion book to The Bullworker Bible™. Both books are approved by the makers of The Bullworker®. Each week has a detailed note section, suggestions about exercise days, and rest times etc. so you know exactly what to do, and when to do it. The course can be used with the Bullworker® Classic, the Steel Bow®, the Bullworker X5, the Bully Extreme, the ISO 7x, and the Bullworker X7. The course contains alternative/extra exercises using the Iso-Bow® and the Bow Extension® to increase the range and effectiveness of The Bullworker®. Required equipment: Bullworker® Classic, or a similar device. Recommended equipment: Steel Bow®, Bow Extension® kit, 2 x Iso-Bows®.

The Bullworker Compendium™ - The Bullworker Bible™ and The Bullworker90™ Course Combined

This book has been approved by **TWiEA** – The World Isometric Exercise Association (www.TWiEA.com).

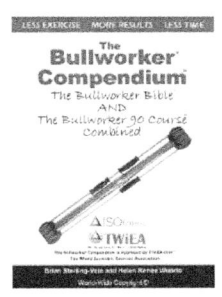

At over 570+ pages The Bullworker Compendium™ is the combination of both The Bullworker Bible™ and The Bullworker 90™ Course in a single huge book.   To save printing costs the only thing we have eliminated are duplicated sections, everything else remains the same.   This way we can offer both books in one for less than the combined price of the two other books.   The Bullworker Compendium™ starts with The Bullworker Bible™, and at the end of that, it progresses seamlessly into The Bullworker 90™ Course.

The Doorway to Strength™ - Turn a Door into a Strength-Building Multigym

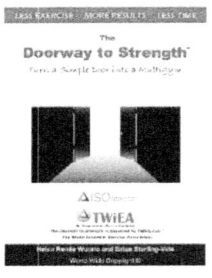

This book has been approved by **TWiEA** – The World Isometric Exercise Association (www.TWiEA.com).

The Doorway to Strength™ shows how a simple door, doorway, and doorframe can be used to create a multi-gym of exercises using the amazing Iso-Bow® exerciser. It demonstrates how to perform a host of powerful and effective isometric exercises such as the door leg press and shoulder power push, together with many other exercises to work all the major body parts. Required equipment: 2 x Iso-Bows® (preferably 4), a solid door and frame, and a door wedge/stop.

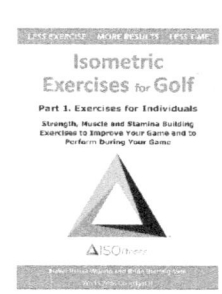

Isometric Exercises for Golf™ Part 1. Exercises for Individuals

This book has been approved by **TWiEA** – The World Isometric Exercise Association (www.TWiEA.com).

There is no such thing as a quick game of golf which means that there is not always enough spare time to exercise in a gym as well as play golf. A series of advanced 7 to 10-second isometric exercises either while you play, or practice is the answer. Perform just one isometric exercise at each hole and at the end of an 18-hole game you have completed a powerful total-body workout. The average golf club is a perfect Improvised Isometric Exercise Device or IIED, so you are carrying your go-anywhere multi-gym everywhere you play. Golf pros and coaches can also use these exercises as a handy resource to practice with their clients. Part 1. is a resource guide of isometric exercises that can be performed as an individual. Note: The exercises in this book are either the same or similar to those in our books: Nordic Walking or Trekking Pole. However, the Isometric Exercises for Golf book 1 contains some special exercises designed to increase the strength and power of your golf swing.

Isometric Exercises for Golf™ Part 2. Exercises for Partner-Pairs

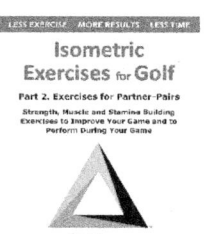

This book has been approved by **TWiEA** – The World Isometric Exercise Association (www.TWiEA.com).

This is the companion to Book 1 and is entirely focussed on exercises that are best performed in partnered pairs, with a buddy at any time during a break, a game, or during practice sessions.

Isometric Exercises for Nordic Walking and Trekking™ - Part 1. Exercises for Individuals

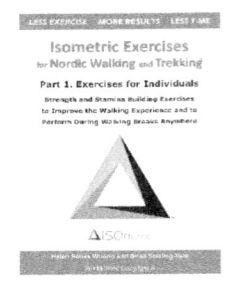

This book has been approved by **TWiEA** – The World Isometric Exercise Association (www.TWiEA.com).

Strength and Stamina Building Exercises to Improve the Walking Experience and to Perform During Walking Breaks Anywhere. More Nordic Walkers and Trekkers than ever before perform proven gym-quality isometric exercise routines to exercise their whole body during scheduled walk breaks in almost any location. This book, Part 1. is an exercise resource guide of isometric exercises that can be performed as an individual, either outdoors or at home. Note: The exercises in this book are either the same or similar to those in our other books using a golf club. However, the Isometric Exercises for Golf book 1 contains some special exercises designed to increase the strength and power of your golf swing.

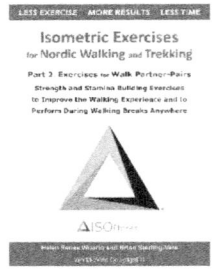

Isometric Exercises for Nordic Walking and Trekking™ - Part 2. Exercises for Walk Partner-Pairs

This book has been approved by **TWiEA** – The World Isometric Exercise Association (www.TWiEA.com).

This is the companion to Book 1 and is entirely focussed on exercises that are best performed as a partner-pair, with a buddy at any time during a walking break anywhere.

The Sixty Second ASS Workout™ - The Ultimate 60-Second Workout to Shape, Tone, Lift, and Give You the Backside You've Always Wanted

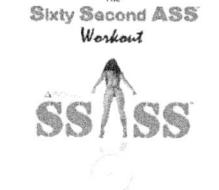

This book has been approved by **TWiEA** – The World Isometric Exercise Association (www.TWiEA.com).

The Sixty Second ASS Workout™, or SSASS™ workout, is the fastest and most effective "ass" workout ever devised. Scientifically proven advanced isometric exercises deliver a no-nonsense time-efficient workout that does everything you need to make your ass tight, firm, shapely and strong. No more time-wasting workouts where you twist, shake, wiggle around that might be fun but never deliver the results you want. Everyone has 60 seconds to spare, even on the busiest day, so, you are just 60 seconds a day from having a great ass. Required Equipment: 2 x Iso-Bows available on Amazon or from Bullworker.com

The Zero-Footprint Isolation Lockdown Workout

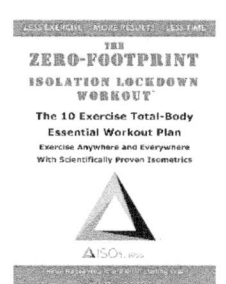

The 10 Exercise Total-Body Essential Workout Plan Exercise Anywhere and Everywhere With Scientifically Proven Isometrics

This book has been approved by TWiEA – The World Isometric Exercise Association (www.TWiEA.com). In 2020, the world changed forever due to The Coronavirus COVID-19 global pandemic. Gyms are typically some of the unhealthiest of places when it comes to virus and disease transmissions were suddenly forced to close. Immediately, millions of people who loved to exercise regularly were forced to learn how to exercise at home, sometimes in extremely confined spaces. Science had also shown that people who trained for long periods and especially endurance athletes were more susceptible to illness and especially upper respiratory tract infections which is where the killer COVID-19 strikes. The Zero-Footprint Isolation Lockdown Workout™ delivers the 10-essential total-body isometric exercises that can be performed in the smallest of spaces. If you can stand and sit, then you can perform a powerful workout routine in as little as 70 seconds a day!

Improvised Isometric Exercise Devices - The Daisy Chain - How a Simple Climber's Daisy Chain Can Become a Powerful Improvised Isometric Exercise Device or IIED

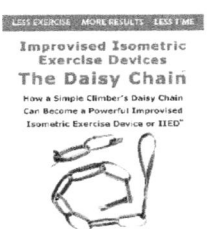

This book has been approved by TWiEA – The World Isometric Exercise Association (www.TWiEA.com).

If you want to add some equipment to your workout, then it does not have to be expensive or proprietary. Improvised Isometric Exercise Devices or IIEDs come in all shapes and sizes and are only limited by your imagination and knowledge of good biomechanics. Basic climbing equipment can also become extremely powerful IIEDs. One of the most effective is the powerful and extremely versatile daisy chain. This book is a valuable resource listing many improvised isometric exercises that can be performed with a daisy chain. It also tells you how they can be effectively used, adapted, safely extended and it gives you some essential information about daisy chains, their strength, and their construction.

Improvised Isometric Exercise Devices - The Climber's Sling - How a Simple Climber's Sling Can Become a Powerful Improvised Isometric Exercise Device or IIED

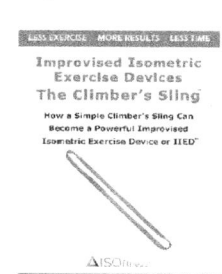

This book has been approved by TWiEA – The World Isometric Exercise Association (www.TWiEA.com).

If you want to add some equipment to your workout, then it does not have to be expensive or proprietary. Improvised Isometric Exercise Devices or IIEDs come in all shapes and sizes and are only limited by your imagination and knowledge of good biomechanics. Basic climbing equipment can also become extremely powerful IIEDs. One of the most effective is the powerful and extremely versatile climber's sling. This book is a valuable resource listing many improvised isometric exercises that can be performed with a climber's sling. It also tells you how they can be effectively used, adapted, safely extended and it gives you some essential information about climber's slings, their strength, and their construction.

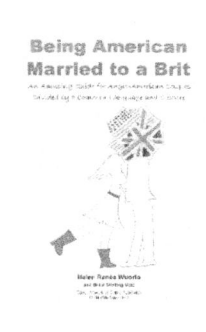

Being American Married to a Brit™ - An Amusing Guide for Anglo-American Couples Divided by a Common Language and Culture

When I first started dating my British man, I never gave a second thought about differences in language and culture. Why would I? After all, we

Americans speak English, or do we...? As dating quickly turned into an engagement and then being married to my British gentleman, I found that our common language and culture was a quirky, eye-opening, and highly amusing roller-coaster ride. At times during the most basic every-day conversations, I would be listening to his words with glazed eyes, wondering what on earth he was saying. It was as if we were both speaking a completely different language, even though the words that comprised the language were the same. I decided to write this book and dedicate it to all transatlantic couples who will regularly find themselves completely divided and confused by their common language and culture.

Mental Martial Arts™ - intellectual Life and Business Combat Skills

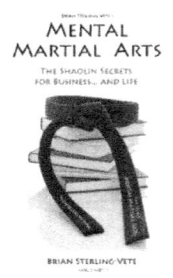

Brian Sterling-Vete's Mental Martial Arts is a system of intellectual life-combat skills using the tactics and principles of the physical martial arts. All interaction in life, in business, and when communicating with others is simply an exchange of energy, power and influence. Each party is always exerting maximum influence over the other to gain the outcome they prefer. The more powerful and persuasive will usually win unless the apparently 'weaker' person is trained in the Mental Martial Arts. You can learn how to verbally, intellectually, and emotionally guide, channel, and redirect the energy of others, even powerful people, and large organisations to more frequently achieve the outcome that you desire in life and business. It also contains a section about how to handle a potentially hostile media in the event of a crisis where the experience Brian gained in over a decade with BBC TV News and a lifetime in the martial arts can help you and your organisation stay Media Safe. www.mentalmartialarts.tv

Tuxedo Warriors™

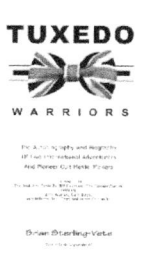

Tuxedo Warriors is the companion book to both The Tuxedo Warrior book and the movie. These books are the biography and autobiography of the iconic cult author, composer, moviemaker Cliff Twemlow. The original book ended at the beginning of what has been called by many 'the Golden Age' of Video Cinematography which Cliff Twemlow inspired. Tuxedo Warriors continues the story from the point when Cliff's original book finishes, and it is the most complete biography of Cliff Twemlow ever written. It is also the autobiography Brian Sterling-Vete who played a central role in this unique, entertaining, and true story of two 'Renaissance-Men' and their adventures as guerrilla moviemakers.

The Tuxedo Warrior™ by Cliff Twemlow – Prologue and epilogue by Brian Sterling-Vete.

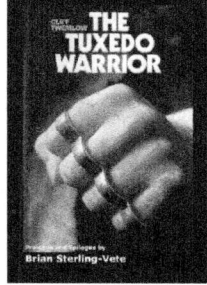

There are many ways in which a Doorman can gain respect. Numerous methods applied to the principal. In my profession, every available technique must be utilised, depending on the situation and circumstances. Would-be

transgressors either move-off the premises quietly acknowledging your diplomatic approach. Or, the other alternative whereby physical persuasion must be exercised, which either quells their pugilistic desires or it triggers their aggressive instincts, turning the whole incident into a bloody and violent encounter. 'The Tuxedo Warrior,' pulls no punches in its brawling, savage, colourful, and entertaining exposure of society's nightlife activities.

The above is the original text from the rear cover of Cliff's book. Where Cliff's original book finishes, my own book 'Tuxedo Warriors' begins to complete Cliff's colourful life story. I am honoured to be friends with Cliff's eldest son, Barry, and sincerely thank him for enabling this book and the others that Cliff wrote to be re-published.

Paranormal Investigation - The Black Book of Scientific Ghost Hunting and How to Investigate Paranormal Phenomena™

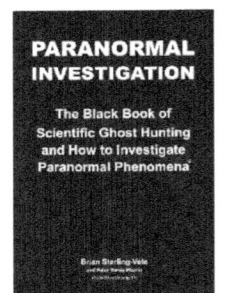

This book is ideal for those who are new to paranormal investigation and ghost hunting, and for more experienced investigators who want to learn more about how to apply a critical-path scientific approach. It contains a special scientific critical path graphic page to work from when devising ghost hunting experiments and to help train team members. There is a step-by-step guide to a complete paranormal investigation and vital information about how to protect yourself from malevolent paranormal entities that can attack you. It also contains ideas for potentially paranormally active and 'haunted' locations and several accounts of previously untold paranormal events including the remarkable Redwood Falls Minnesota UFO sighting.

The Pike™ by Cliff Twemlow – Prologue and epilogue by Brian Sterling-Vete.

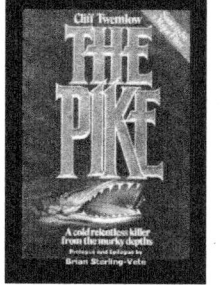

ITS FIRST VICTIMS - A screeching swan... A fisherman overboard... A drunken woman...

One by one, the mysterious killer in Lake Windermere claims its terrified victims. Tearing off limbs with its monstrous teeth, horribly mutilating bodies. Fear sweeps the peaceful holiday resort when experts identify the creature as a giant pike.... A hellish creature with the strength to rupture boats, and the anger to attack them. But for some, the terror becomes a bonanza—the traders who cater to the gathering crowds of ghouls on the shore. And, they will do anything to stop divers finding the creature. Meanwhile the ripples of bloodshed widen.... The Pike.

The above is the original text from the rear cover of Cliff's book which was to become a movie in the early 1980s starring Joan Collins.

The Beast of Kane™ by Cliff Twemlow – Prologue and epilogue by Brian Sterling-Vete.

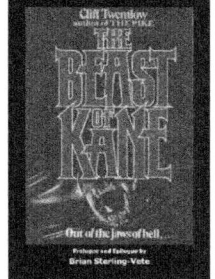

When the Gordon Family open their door to a stray Elkhound, they unwittingly welcome-in the forces of evil. For, according to the local priest, the huge dog is Satan himself, fulfilling an ancient prophecy. But, no one will believe this warning... Even when sheep – and wolves – are mysteriously slaughtered. Even when frenzied pets turn on their owners. Even when Emily Forrest is savagely eaten alive – the first of many human victims. As winter tightens its icy grip on the remote town of Kane, its unprotected people must face an unearthly terror.

The above is the original text from the rear cover of Cliff's book. This was the first of Cliff's books to be accepted by Hammer Film Studios to be made into a big-screen horror movie, along with Cliff's other book, The Pike.

The Haunting of Lilford Hall™ - The Birthplace of the United States as a Nation Haunted by the Man Behind The Pilgrim Fathers

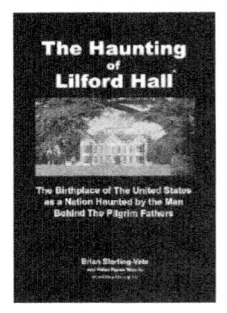

The Haunting of Lilford Hall is one of the most baffling cases ever recorded of paranormal activity experienced simultaneously by multiple people.

Between 2012 and 2013, a team of 13 people came together to produce a historical TV documentary, not a paranormal investigation. The TV documentary was about the life of Robert Browne, the man who was behind The Pilgrim Fathers sailing on The Mayflower to settle the first civilian colony on the American continent. Without Robert Browne, there may never have been the United States of America, at least not as we know it today.

They experienced doors that refused to stay closed, they had debris thrown at them, they had a door silently ripped away from the hinges and doorframe while they were in the next room. There were even several recorded multi-witness apparitions of a man fitting Robert Browne's recorded description. It is believed by many that the ghost of Robert Browne, the "Grandfather" of the United States as a nation, still haunts Lilford Hall to this day.

- Robert Browne was the man who separated church from state in the reign of Queen Elizabeth 1st which is the underpinning of the United States.
- Robert Browne's words are written into the constitution of the United States.
- Robert Browne's direct descendent officially fired the first shot in the American war of independence.
- Robert Browne's beloved Lilford Hall estate was the home of President George Washington's Mother.
- Robert Browne's beloved Lilford Hall estate was the home of President Quincy Adams' family.

www.MajorVision.com

Printed in Great Britain
by Amazon